Why People Don't Heal

and How They Can

Also by Caroline Myss

Anatomy of the Spirit

The Creation of Health
(with C. Norman Shealy, M.D., Ph.D.)

WHY PEOPLE DON'T HEAL

◆

AND HOW THEY CAN

CAROLINE MYSS, Ph.D.

BANTAM BOOKS
SYDNEY • AUCKLAND • TORONTO • NEW YORK • LONDON

Grateful acknowledgement is made to the following for permission
to reprint previously published material: Ballantine Books for poetry
from the *Tao Te Ching*, translated by Robert Henricks. Copyright ©
1989 by Robert Henricks. Reprinted by permission of Ballantine
Books, a division of Random House, Inc. Princeton University Press
for permission to reprint "Seven Power Centers or Chakras of the
Kundalini System" from *Mythic Image* by Joseph Campbell.
Copyright © 1974 by Princeton University press. Reprinted by
permission of Princeton University Press.

First Published by Harmony Books, a division of Crown Publishers,
Inc., 201 East 50th Street, New York, New York 10022

Designed by June Bennett-Tantillo

Library of Congress Cataloguing-in-Publication Data
Myss, Caroline M.
Why people don't heal and how they can / Caroline Myss. - 1st ed.
p.   cm.
Includes bibliographical references and index.
1. Medicine and psychology. 2. Mind and body. 3. Medicine,
Psychosomatic. 4. Personality–Health aspects. I. Title.
R726.5.M98   1997
610'.1'9-dc21   97-22798
                                                     CIP

ISBN 0 73380 203 6

Bantam books are published by

Transworld Publishers (Aust) Pty Limited
15-25 Helles Ave, Moorebank, NSW 2170
Transworld Publishers (NZ) Pty Limited
3 William Pickering Drive, Albany, Auckland
Transworld Publishers (UK) Limited
61-63 Uxbridge Road, Ealing,
London W5 5SA
Bantam Doubleday Dell Publishing Group Inc
1540 Broadway, New York, New York 10036

Printed by McPherson's Printing Group, Maryborough, Victoria
10 9 8 7 6 5 4 3 2

This book is dedicated to
Rachel Naomi Remen, M.D.,
and Daniel Lowenstein, M.D.—
with great love and appreciation
for having come into my life.

Contents

✦

Introduction:
What Is Energy Medicine?

✦

M y intention in writing this book is to offer readers a new perspective on health, specifically on why we don't heal and how we can. I may seem to be entering the subject of healing through the back door, since I am giving so much attention to why we fail to heal, but I believe that many of us are almost as afraid of healing as we are of illness. By understanding how fear and other negative emotions adversely affect healing, you may more easily identify how you are interfering, consciously or unconsciously, with your own healing process.

It has become apparent to me that assuming that everyone wants to heal is both misleading and potentially dangerous. Illness can, for instance, become a powerful way to get attention you might not otherwise receive—as a form of leverage, illness can seem almost attractive. Illness may also convey the message that you have to change your life quite drastically. Because change is among the most frightening aspects of life, you may fear change more intensely than illness and enter into a pattern of postponing the changes you need to make.

A central misconception of today's holistic culture is the belief that all illness results from personal negativity, either from tragic past experiences, from negative attitudes that contaminate our minds and bodies, or from bad past-life karma. Yet negativity is not the only source of illness: It can also emerge as the answer to a prayer. It can physically guide us onto a path of insight and learning upon which we would otherwise never have set foot. It may be a catalyst for expanding personal consciousness as well as for understanding the greater meaning of life.

As terrifying as disease is, it is also an invitation to enter into the nature of mystery. Our lives are made up of a series of mysteries that we are meant to explore but that are meant to remain unsolved. We are meant to live with the questions we have about our lives, even use them as companions, and allow them to lead us into the deepest recesses of our nature, wherein we discover the Sacred. I hope that this book will help you find new ways of framing the meaning of illness and other life challenges and help you move deeper into your mysteries and further along your personal path toward spiritual mastery.

While illness can help you find your essential sacredness, your oneness with God, humanity, and all living creatures, you don't have to become ill in order to begin to understand your spirit and heal your life. I find that people begin to see and understand themselves as sacred through learning about what I call energy medicine. According to energy medicine, the human spirit is a manifestation of energy. We all have seven energy centers in our bodies, which in the Hindu system are called chakras. Each chakra roughly corresponds to a location in the physical body. I like to think of the chakras as "energetic" computer disks or data banks that collect information of all sorts. In my work I have discovered that these seven energy centers correspond to the various life issues and challenges with which the seven sacraments of Christianity and the ten sefirot of the Tree of Life in the Jewish Kabbalistic tradition are also meant to help us.

Our spirit grows into maturity and increasing self-understanding through seven stages of spiritual development. As we progress through these stages, we gain different kinds of personal power. The chakras—and their counterparts in the sacraments and

the Tree of Life—mark an inner path of spiritual evolution. They
form the steps on an unfolding of our personal path toward awakening a higher consciousness. Learning the language of the chakras
and nurturing these spiritual qualities can simultaneously strengthen
our physical bodies and help us heal illness or maintain health.

A man named Ben, who came to one of my workshops while
dealing with prostate cancer, responded instantly when I explained
the correspondences between the chakras, the sacraments, and the
Tree of Life. For him, they formed a new language of healing. Ben
went on to use the imagery from the workshop, which I also teach
in this book, continually in his own healing. Whenever he visited
his doctor for treatment, he said a prayer or mantra beforehand in
which he invoked the power of the chakras, sacraments, and Tree
of Life to "activate" his body. Within six months his cancer went
into remission.

As a medical intuitive, I describe for people the nature of
their physical diseases as well as the energetic dysfunctions that
are present within their bodies. I read the energy field that permeates and surrounds the body, picking up information about
dramatic childhood experiences, behavior patterns, even superstitious beliefs, all of which have bearing on the person's physical
health. Based on the information I perceive intuitively in their
energy fields, including the chakras, I can make recommendations
for treating their condition on both a physical and spiritual level.

The intention behind using energy medicine is to treat the
body and the spirit equally. As you learn the language of the
chakras, you will come to recognize the emotional, psychological,
and spiritual stress factors that affect your health and that correspond to your physical symptoms. Your health is also affected by
your self-esteem and relationship history, your response to profound or traumatic experiences or memories, and your energy
management in everyday situations.

Energy medicine is actually quite an old field of knowledge;
its principles and techniques were certainly known to the ancient
Hindu, Chinese, and shamanic healers. What I believe is new is

my correlation of Eastern spiritual ideas of the chakras with Western spiritual truths and ethics to create a new language of energy. The word *energy* has taken on a number of meanings recently, but I use it to refer to both physical and spiritual energy. Eastern metaphysics and Western Theosophy have variously described a series of energetic sheaths or layers surrounding and interacting with the physical body. When mystics tell us that we are much vaster than we know, part of what they are talking about is this energy field. Everyone has such an energy field, and it contains valuable information about their physical, psychological, and spiritual condition and needs.

As an intuitive, I can read this field and see an actual connection between, say, the loss of energy in the pancreas and the creation of diabetes or hypoglycemia. I can also track that development to specific issues in a person's life—for example, to the stress resulting from too much responsibility or the fear of it. And by learning the language of the chakras, you too can, I believe, become more adept at seeing physical and spiritual energy connections and using this perception to prevent or heal illness by making certain life changes.

You can also learn to use Symbolic sight, to intuitively interpret the power symbols in your life, to reveal where you have invested your personal energy, to uncover the greater meaning of your life's challenges apart from the literal events, and to discover how this all connects to your health.

This book gives a short course in the language of the chakras, shorter than in my previous book, *Anatomy of the Spirit*, so that you will have an easy reference to the language of energy to begin your own course of healing. If you have read *Anatomy of the Spirit* or *The Creation of Health*, you can use the review of the chakras as a refresher. The chakras are vertically aligned from the base of the spine to the crown of the head, suggesting that we ascend toward the Divine by gradually mastering the seductive pull of the material world. At each stage we gain a more refined understanding of personal and spiritual power, since each chakra represents a spiritual life-lesson or challenge common to all human beings. Although the chakra system was developed in the East and served as the basis for certain Hindu, Buddhist, and Taoist teachings, the kinds of energy they describe are congruent with the energy defined by the sefirot of the Kabbalah and are meant to be managed by the Christian sacraments.

I review the language of the chakras both at the beginning of the book and more extensively at the end. I include ways to use their energy for healing, and techniques for developing Symbolic sight, and I also present a larger symbolic context for healing. Although I have not written about this concept before, I have been using it in my workshops for some time now. Simply put, I see the history of our spiritual development as a succession of power (or energy) cultures that roughly correspond to several astrological ages. An astrological age lasts about two thousand years, during which time human consciousness develops in new ways. During each of these ages, a certain kind of energy was dominant, and it affected people's lives, health, and spiritual outlook. Each age has contributed to human knowledge distinct perceptions about the nature of reality and the power of the human spirit—perceptions that still affect our health and souls today. To help understand the kind of power or energy most characteristic of these ages, I enlist the symbolism of astrology.

The age of Aries ran from around 2,000 B.C. to the birth of Christ, which introduced the Piscean age. And as anyone familiar with the musical *Hair!* already knows, we are now entering the age of Aquarius. Aries, a fire sign, represents the fire of ignition, of initial creation, of the beginning of the zodiac itself and, as I see it, a revving up of many cultures and civilizations. A unity of Tribal culture, thought, and law began in the Arien age, which superseded the more primitive Tribalism of the preceding age of Taurus. Aries was an era of dominating the physical environment, of laws from Hammurabi to Moses, of laying the social and cultural foundations on which we based the emotional, psychological, and spiritual development of the next era.

The Piscean age was a time of dualism, when human consciousness divided in a powerful way into polarities, such as those between Western and Eastern culture, church and state, body and spirit (in a split epitomized by Manicheanism), the science of magnetics, even political polarities of left and right. At the same time, we broke away from the Tribal mind to develop a clearer sense of self: the Renaissance celebrated the individual, artists and composers began to sign their work, and people began keeping diaries. The concept of law evolved from tribal codes to the rights of the individual as embodied in the Magna Carta, the U.S. Constitution, and more recent laws aimed at loosening social and religious restrictions.

As we enter the age of Aquarius at the end of the twentieth century, we are moving from astrological eras represented by fish and animals into one symbolized by a human being: the water-bearer. If division was the theme of Pisces, wholeness is the theme of Aquarius, in which we are striving to discover a spiritual unity. The religions of the world have begun to try to accommodate each other in unprecedented ways, and we appear to have developed a global marketplace, global technology, and global awareness of social justice and the need for environmental preservation despite obvious breaches of both. The chant first voiced at the 1968 Democratic Convention in Chicago, "The whole world is watching!" has become as prophetic as Marshall McLuhan's description of the emerging world culture as a "global village." This new kind of worldwide tribal unity will replace the much more limited tribalism of the Arien age.

With each astrological age, spiritual consciousness has matured to include a greater awareness of ourselves, of the spirit inherent in other life, and of the greater power around us. We need to examine the role that each of these eras has played so we can understand how we have absorbed their attitudes and beliefs and how and where they are hampering our efforts to heal ourselves individually, physically, and spiritually. As the astrological ages progressed, they encompassed a succession of different mindsets and different kinds of physical and spiritual power. I have labeled these attitudes and powers Tribal, Individual, and Symbolic. Understanding the characteristics of power inherent in each astrological age transfers to the ability to recognize that we have multiple capacities for perception; Tribal sight is fine sensory; Individual sight extends into emotional and psychological interpretation, which adds relativity to perception; and Symbolic sight reaches into the impersonal realm of archetypal sight. Tribal power, characteristic of the age of Aries, is essentially group consciousness, identified most strongly to membership in a family, ethnic group, religion, and nation. The strengths of Tribal power—security, order, loyalty, a sense of identity—can easily become its weaknesses—rigidity, conformity, patriarchalism, xenophobia. Tribal consciousness focuses on externals to the exclusion of many internal individual and spiritual needs, and thus is essentially a fine sensory perceptual system.

Individual power, by contrast, is related to our emotional and psychological identity epitomized by the Piscean age, during which science and the arts flourished and the value of individual genius ascended. The weaknesses of Individual power are excessive focus on the self, narcissism, and the tendency to polarize good and evil, male and female, East and West, knowledge and intuition, left brain and right brain.

Finally, Symbolic power is that which allows us to see things in impersonal terms, to view both history and our own lives with the overarching, unifying vision characteristic of the Aquarian age, which is calling on us to discover the inner power of consciousness. The energy of this emergent astrological age pulls us to create a culture in which spirit and energy have a higher priority than matter and the body, and to understand that the energy within our minds, bodies, and spirits is the same as that of God or the greater divinity. As we enter the Aquarian age, however, we remain connected to the evolutionary energy contained in each previous age.

The ability to think of power and energy in these three ways helps us gain an entirely new perception of our individual life choices, how they affect our spirit and health, and how we can help ourselves recover our health and call back our spirits.

In the grand scope and clash of human history can be seen a reflection of our own spiritual development and our own need to adapt to change. Difficulties and illness are a necessary part of our spiritual evolution. Just as we look back at world history and create meaning from seemingly unconnected events, so can we create meaning out of disruptions and challenges in our daily lives.

My intention, and my hope, is that the blending of all this information will provide readers with a means through which they can enter illness without fear and face change with courage. I hope that this book will provide you with some new and beneficial methods of seeing yourself, your health challenge, and your healing potential. I particularly want you to re-envision yourself in the context of today's culture, so that you can develop a way of seeing yourself Symbolically. By so doing, I believe, you can ignite the healing fire that lies in wait deep within the human spirit, which will guide you to the right healing steps for you to take.

The healing fire that has gripped us as individuals is also at work everywhere on the planet, human beings are being compelled by a force much greater than ourselves to heal ourselves, our cultures, our environment—in short, to become a conscious species. This is the reason so many of us desire to be healthy and conscious—and are tormented by our inability to fully reach that goal. Perhaps by understanding the dynamics of this new culture of which we are now a part, we will be more able to become healthy human beings and so begin to fulfill our destiny.

As I have taught people who were trying to heal the Symbolic language of the chakras, sacraments, Tree of Life, and the cultural context to personal healing, I have seen it reinforce a belief in Divine guidance. Developing a fluency in these metaphysical symbols seems to help them make contact with the healing energy inherent in their own spirit.

I met Ellie four years ago in a workshop in Europe, at a time when I was already deeply absorbed by the similarities among the sacraments, the Tree of Life, and the chakra system. I had no idea that Ellie would be the first person with whom I would share this information. In a private conversation, she told me that she had a history of repeated experiences with cancer, beginning eight years before. Her first tumor had shown up in her left leg. It was a small malignant tumor, but following her surgery to have it removed, she was told that it was contained and that all looked well. About four years later she discovered another tumor growing in her arm. After surgery she was told that this one, like the previous one, seemed to be contained, except that her physician now advised her to keep a close watch over her body. At the time of our meeting, Ellie was dealing with her third tumor, which had shown up once again in her leg, three years after her second one. She knew that this one was also malignant, and she was now in a state of total terror that no matter what she did, she could not break her pattern of repeatedly producing malignant tumors. Furthermore, she had become obsessed with fear that every pain she experienced in her body, no matter where it might be, was an indication that another tumor was growing.

Ellie was deeply perplexed, because she knew that she was doing all the right things to keep her body clean. If diet, exercise, therapy, yoga, and holistic treatments of every variety were not working, what else was there for her to do? Was there a God who truly listened, and if so, where was this God in her life?

There have been several times in my work when I have felt myself at a loss for the right words, and this was one of them. For lack of anything else to say, I shared with Ellie that I had often asked the same questions and had never had the answer come in a way I had anticipated. I told her that as I worked with clients, using the chakra system as my only reference point, I frequently felt that the model, while ancient and sacred, was incomplete. Then one day, as I was teaching a group of students, I looked at the model of seven circles that I had drawn on the board, and instead of seeing the chakra system, I found myself thinking about the seven Christian sacraments. Shortly afterward I had a similar intuition about the Tree of Life as described in the Jewish Kabbalah. I was struck with the wonderment over the union of these three sacred traditions and the realization that the voice of the Divine was showing me the holy passage of sacred energy through the human body.

I described for Ellie the union of these three spiritual traditions and added that their merger needed to be viewed through a Symbolic lens to tap into their power. I asked her to interpret Baptism, the first sacrament, as representing her ability to see her entire life and all the people in it, along with her relationship with this earth itself, as a gift that she has been asked to accept. I suggested that she add to that not only the meaning of Shekhinah, representing a union with the community of humanity, but also the energy of Gaia—the life-force of Nature itself. As I spoke to Ellie, she closed her eyes, and I could sense her intently following my words. I told her to feel this connection to the earth and to her life and to direct it into her first chakra, with the image that she was reconnecting fully to the system of life.

I continued this description through the remaining chakras, and by the time I had finished, Ellie appeared to be in a deep state of meditation. She emerged about half an hour later and spoke calmly. "I didn't realize that the consequence of my bouts with cancer was destroying more than my body," she said. "I didn't realize that I had completely lost touch with the energy of life itself, and that no amount of nutrition can replace that. I need to heal my connection to life and not just focus on healing cancer."

Ellie repeated that visualization constantly. She stayed in touch with me, and with each phone call she reported feeling her physical system returning to life. She said that she had created a structure to her visualizations in which she worked to incorporate the meaning of the lessons inherent in each chakra, sacrament, and sefira of the Tree of Life. She decided to postpone her surgery for a while because she wanted to see if her internal work could actually produce a change in her physical body. If it could, then she would know that she had finally broken her cycle of cancer.

Within a month, her tumor began to show signs of shrinking, which was the signal Ellie had been waiting for. She had it surgically removed, believing to the depths of her soul that she would never again have a recurrence of cancer.

Although Ellie's is a particuarly dramatic healing of a physical disease, keep in mind that healings can occur for many different kinds of ailments and can also be emotional and spiritual as well as physical. The stories you will read in this book range from the everyday to the extraordinary with many gradations in between, and you are likely to see your own health challenge or life crisis reflected in one or more of them. I want you to feel confident that there is something here that will facilitate your healing.

One of the main beliefs that I want you to adopt in order to heal your life or illness is a belief in the importance of forgiveness. Forgiveness frees up the energy necessary for healing. I will present suggestions on how to go about forgiving—or letting go of—the past, and will give you new rituals and invocations for helping you see your present life Symbolically, bolster your personal energy, connect you with Divine energy, and help you heal.

Although the first half of this book treats in depth the reasons why people don't heal, the second half will show you in detail how you can. We'll begin by discussing what I consider to be the greatest stumbling block to healing in our culture today.

Part One

✦

WHY
PEOPLE
DON'T
HEAL . . .

Chapter One

◆

WOUNDOLOGY AND
THE HEALING FIRE

In the late spring of 1988, I arrived at the Findhorn Community in northeastern Scotland to teach a healing workshop. At that point in my career the people who came to my workshops had tended to be searching for a personal healing. They expected me, as a medical intuitive, to facilitate their healing directly by giving them an individual reading and setting up a treatment regimen for them. (These days my workshops are largely filled with self-reliant people who want to learn how to become more intuitive by learning to "speak chakras" and so heal themselves and their lives, or professionals looking to learn how to help others heal.)

Though I myself am not a healer, I was happy to help them, of course, to the best of my abilities. Often in my readings I was simply validating the suspicions, insights, or intuitions that they already had about themselves and the changes they needed to make in their lives. Sometimes these readings ignited an inner physical and spiritual healing process. Even so, at that time, my workshop participants and I all felt that we were on the right track. After all, healing and health had become the main focus of the holistic or consciousness culture as well as the center of my life. Almost everyone I met, professionally and personally, spoke about either wanting to become a healer or needing a healer, being on their way to visit a new healer, or believing that they were meant to be a healer as soon as they had completed their own healing.

I enjoyed traveling around the world and meeting spiritually committed people who needed me as much as I needed them, and I had especially come to love Findhorn, a community of about three hundred people sharing an organic, cooperative life and a respect for all spiritual paths. Some of the community members reside in an enchanting, converted turn-of-the-century hotel; others have made their home quarters in a beautiful park area alongside the Findhorn Bay. The rugged beauty of the Scottish Highlands, combined with the spiritual focus of the community, make Findhorn a most attractive place to be. Whenever I go there, I seem to receive a special energetic charge that results in some important insight, and this visit in 1988 was no exception. This time, however, the insight came in a rather unlikely way.

Prior to beginning the weeklong workshop, I had arranged to have lunch with my dear friend Mary. Having arrived early in the dining room, I joined two gentlemen for tea. Mary entered a while later, and when she walked over to our table, I introduced her to my companions. She had just extended her hand to greet them when another member of the Findhorn community, Wayne, came up to her and asked, "Mary, are you busy on June eighth? We're looking for someone to escort a guest coming to Findhorn for the day."

The tone of Mary's response was as revealing as its length. She snapped, "June eighth? Did you say June eighth?" Suffused with anger and resentment, she continued, "Absolutely not! June eighth is my incest support group meeting, and I would never, ever miss that meeting! We count on each other, after all. We incest victims have to be there for one another. I mean, who else do we have?"

Mary went on for a while longer, but this is as much as I can accurately remember. I was captivated by the instantaneous dramatics triggered by a simple question about her schedule. Wayne hardly took notice of her response, thanked her, and left, but I was astonished. Later, as Mary and I were having lunch, I asked her about her behavior:

"Mary, why, when you were answering Wayne's question about your schedule, did you have to let all three men know that you had suffered incest as a young girl, that you were still angry about it, that you were angry with men in general, and that you intended to control the atmosphere of the conversation with your anger? All Wayne asked you was, 'Are you busy June eighth?' and in response you gave these three men a miniature therapy class. A simple yes or no would have done fine."

Mary looked at me as if I had betrayed her. Her body stiffened, and she emphasized her words in an ice-cold, defensive tone: "I answered that way because I am a victim of incest." She drew back from the table, stopped eating, and threw her napkin over her plate, indicating that our lunch together had come to a close. Although I didn't realize it at that moment, so had our friendship.

"Mary, honey," I replied, softening my own tone somewhat, "I know you're a victim of incest, but what I'm trying to figure out is why you found it necessary to tell two strangers and Wayne your history when all he wanted to know was whether you could help out on June eighth. Did you want these men to treat you a certain way or talk to you in a certain way? What made you lay your wounds out on the table within seven seconds of meeting two new people?"

Mary told me that I simply did not understand because I had not endured what she and numerous other incest victims had gone through, but that she had expected me as a friend to be more compassionate. I replied that lack of compassion had nothing to do with what I was asking her. I could feel the separation of energy between us as I realized that in order for our friendship to continue, I needed to "speak wounds" to Mary, to follow some very specific rules of how a supportive friend was to behave, and to bear always in mind that she defined herself by a negative experience.

In addition to her painful childhood history, Mary also had a history of chronic ailments. She was always in pain—some days emotional, some days physical. Though she was kind and always ready to support her friends, she much preferred the company of people who had also had abusive childhoods. That day at our lunch, I realized that Mary needed to be with people who spoke the same language and shared the same mindset and behaviors. I immediately began to think of this attitude as "woundology." I have since become convinced that when we define ourselves by our wounds, we burden and lose our physical and spiritual energy and open ourselves to the risk of illness.

That day I felt as if I had been catapulted out of the surrounding healing culture of Findhorn and the general consciousness movement and was viewing it as an outsider. Although I had not previously noticed this pattern of thought and behavior in Mary or in anyone else, the very next day, curiously, a miniature version of the Mary incident took place in my workshop.

I had arrived twenty minutes early to get ready for my presentation and noticed a woman sitting alone. I sat down next to her and asked, "What's your name?" That's all I asked. Yet without even looking at me, she responded:

"I'm a victim of incest, but I'm fifty-six years old now and I'm over that trauma. I have a wonderful support group, and several of us get together at least once a week, which I believe is essential to healing."

She still had not told me her name, so I asked again, "And what's your name?" But she still didn't answer me directly. She seemed to be in a daze. It felt to me as if she had been preparing for a long time to say something publicly, and now, given the opportunity, she couldn't hear any questions that didn't relate to her agenda. Instead of telling me her name, she said how much she enjoyed coming to workshops like mine because a person was free to speak openly about his or her past, and she hoped that I would allow time for people to share their personal histories. I thanked her and left the room, needing a few moments to gather my thoughts.

Meeting this woman the day after the incident with Mary was not a coincidence. I believe I was being directed to pay attention to the ways we expect to heal our lives—through therapy and support groups. So many people in the midst of a "process" of healing, I saw, are at the same time feeling stuck. They are striving to confront their wounds, valiantly working to bring meaning to terrible past experiences and traumas, and exercising compassionate understanding of others who share their wounds. But they are not healing. They have redefined their lives around their wounds and the process of accepting them. They are not working to get beyond their wounds. In fact, they are stuck in their wounds. Now primed to hear people speak woundology, I believe I was meant to challenge the assumptions that I and many others then held dear—especially the assumption that everyone who is wounded or ill wants the full recovery of their health.

I felt as if I had been given a pair of magical glasses with which to see beneath the behavior of my workshop students. I soon found that the language of woundology was also spoken outside Findhorn. People around the world are confusing the therapeutic value of self-expression with permission to manipulate others with their wounds. Instead of viewing the uncovering of their wounds as an early stage of the healing process, they are using their wounds as a flag and their groups as families and nations.

How did we come to such a pass? A little more than a generation ago, our society was one in which people had difficulty expressing even their most innocent psychological and emotional needs. Today people wear their deepest wounds on their sleeve like a red badge of courage. How did we get to this point? To explain, I have to go back a little further into the past.

OPENING UP

I had begun my work as a medical intuitive in 1983, when I became able to sense illness in other people. At that time I had lacked any training as a health professional, but I had co-founded a publishing company that was dedicated to producing books about consciousness, health, and alternative or complementary medicine. The company published first-person accounts of healings as well as books by more scientifically oriented authors reporting research and discoveries in medical treatments then considered alternative. Those years as both a publisher and a medical intuitive educated me in such complementary ways that I now feel that this personal edification must have been directed by a higher force.

The countless manuscripts we received containing personal stories revealed the depth of fear people feel when facing a terminal illness. But many of the stories also revealed the power of the human spirit to catalyze a healing process that can reclaim the life-force, give meaning to illness, and heal seemingly chronic or terminal diseases. Occasionally I would come across a manuscript by a patient who had lost the battle for physical life but had won an inner tranquillity—a sense of completion of this life and an acceptance of the next stage: the death of the body.

Our culture in the early 1980s was hungry for healing and searching for the experience or state of mind that would ignite a healing fire. When I started to do workshops in 1984, the alternative healing field had established a new vocabulary for psychological and emotional healing. People spoke openly about their physical, mental, and spiritual health. Sharing the details of one's personal history became commonplace, as childhood experiences of incest, molestation, and abuse were openly discussed. The social boundaries that had previously limited acceptable social exchanges had dissolved into a new form of instant intimacy.

This new kind of intimacy grew out of the therapeutic culture of the 1960s. Prior to the 1960s, family secrets, financial information, political affiliations, occupational difficulties, and rumors about who was having an affair with whom were all considered "intimate" information, shared only with family members and very close friends. Even asking someone which presidential candidate he had voted for qualified as a highly intimate question. Nor were such topics discussed easily even among trusted, long-standing intimates: Before the 1960s we lacked the vocabulary for sharing with others the most intimate contents of our emotional lives. Personal emotional needs had not yet been introduced into our general culture. We had not yet become comfortable expressing inner psychological experiences, and our basic physical and emotional needs were generally considered to be met if we took care of our job and family responsibilities.

Moreover, before the 1960s society in general viewed those who sought the help of a psychiatrist as mentally ill. Even in 1972, the revelation that a vice-presidential candidate—George McGovern's running mate, Thomas Eagleton—had undergone psychotherapy was reason enough to have him removed from the ticket. The notion of working through a trauma therapeutically was still unfamiliar, so people viewed any and all mental stress as mental illness. They were afraid of the deeper recesses of the mind and the heart, and few explored them willingly. Those who did acquired reputations as rebels, eccentrics, mystics, hermits, or social outcasts. Most people did not tamper with their internal forces but lived safely within the assumption that if the external parts of their lives were stable, their minds and hearts would naturally attain a degree of contentment.

The therapeutic age gave birth to an entirely new dimension of thought: It opened up the inner world behind our eyes. With each step inward that we took, new perceptions about ourselves emerged and overran the long-guarded boundaries around our emotions and psyches. The concept that "we create our own reality" seemed to spring into popular usage almost out of nowhere. The electric idea that we have a kind of ultimate, personal spiritual power took hold of the popular imagination, and *self-responsibility* became a new power word. We applied these beliefs to every aspect of our lives. Most especially, we began to apply them to the healing process.

People became remarkably eager to "stand and proclaim" not only that they were ill but that they were responsible for their illness, as if this act of public purging in itself contained some kind of power that would guarantee a safe passage into health. In my own workshops and in others I attended, one person after another would describe a particular illness and then add, "I know I'm responsible for this." Where speaking about emotions publicly had once been taboo, it was now a requirement for healing.

Fueled by the notion that an emotional wound that they had previously experienced was at the root of their physical illness, people plunged into their inner lives determined to exorcise every negative memory, thought, and attitude. If they could only unlock that deeply secret emotional impulse, or release that negative childhood experience, they believed, their biological system would respond and reward them with complete health. Almost everyone I encountered during those years was convinced that complete recovery of health was just one psychological insight away. Amazingly enough, every workshop participant who went through this spontaneous public ritual of confession sparkled with enthusiasm and hope. Sometimes, if their story was exceedingly dramatic, applause would follow the confession.

I too believed, as the other workshop participants did, that the psyche held the key to physical healing. An inner power, I was convinced, contained the fuel we needed to reorder our biochemistry and rebuild our bodies. Occasionally someone who had managed to heal an illness—who had not just put the illness into remission but had actually achieved a complete healing—would attain a near-celebrity status at workshops. During the breaks everyone would gather around the self-healer and ask, "What did you do to heal yourself?" I listened, too, eager to learn of some extraordinary treatment, nutritional program, or psychotherapy that would assure a cure.

The self-healers would credit a vast array of factors, including changes in nutrition, vitamin therapy, mud baths, hypnosis, past-life recall, exercise, bodywork, and colon cleansing. Most often, however, they detailed treatments that helped body, mind, and soul together. Regardless of the treatment or the nutritional program that they described, however, the self-healers' greatest gift was the hope they brought to the rest of the group. Those who had made it back to health were considered living proof that individual efforts at self-discovery and healing—that attending workshops, reading books, and learning to express oneself—were bound to pay off.

THE TURNING POINT

For reasons I may never understand, 1988 was the year when views and beliefs about healing shifted, at least within the network in which I was teaching. By this time, I was giving workshops in several different countries, yet that year I encountered the same reaction around the world: Workshop participants were no longer interested solely in how to heal. They wanted to know why they were not healing. They had tried the many healing alternatives available, but they still were not healing. Their focus had shifted from enthusiasm about their individual quest for the right regimen, for the unique combination of mind-body treatments, to a terrible frustration and a ceaseless asking of "What's going on here? Why isn't anything working?"

The desperation they felt was phenomenal. I cannot even begin to recall the number of times I was asked, "Do you think I'm being punished for something?" At that time I had no adequate answer, only the old favorite: "Hold on to your faith, and keep focused on your healing. You can't afford to become negative." This was probably as helpful as saying, "Don't think about a blue monkey." It might even have added to the person's guilt about his or her illness.

To be sure, faith and optimism are important factors in healing any life crisis, including illness, then and now. Back in 1988, however, I could see that people were retreating from the hopefulness of holistic health and self-responsibility and returning to the superstitions of what I call the Tribal mind. They suspected that they were being punished for something awful they had done; they saw the disease or suffering as a judgment of the heavens upon them. Privately, I was becoming as mystified as they were. As I watched them struggle so valiantly with their healing, I too began to wonder if maybe they were doing something wrong, or if maybe they weren't supposed to heal, or if maybe the right treatment hadn't yet been discovered....

THE SEDUCTIVE POWER OF WOUNDS

Then came my fateful luncheon meeting with Mary at Findhorn, followed by my encounter with the incest survivor in my healing workshop, and I began to get an inkling of where the problem lay. For the next few years, woundology became my primary focus. I learned to listen between the lines of what my workshop participants were saying. I began to discern when a person was genuinely going through the specific stage of healing that requires a witness and when someone had discovered the "street" value or social currency of their wound—that is, the manipulative value of the wound.

"Whenever you learn a new word, you should listen carefully," my favorite aunt had taught me as a child, "because you'll hear everyone using it." She was right, and once I tuned in to woundology, the majority of the people in my workshops were conversing in this new language, openly sharing their personal histories with other workshop participants. At times, their sharing even took on a competitive feeling in which one person seemed to attempt to eclipse the painful experiences of another.

The sharing of wounds had become the new language of intimacy, a shortcut to developing trust and understanding. The exchange of intimate revelations, which had been originally developed and intended as appropriate dialogue between therapists and patients, had become the bonding ritual for people just getting to know one another. I met one woman, for instance, who stated upon our introduction that the "rules" of being a friend to her began with agreeing to "honor her wounds." When I asked her to tell me what that meant in practical terms, she said that she was only now beginning to process all of the violations that had happened to her as a child and that in the course of healing these wounds, she would frequently have mood swings and bouts of depression. "Honoring her wounds" meant respecting these moods, not challenging them. She claimed the right to set the tone of any social event of which she was a part. If she was in a "low space," she expected her support system not to introduce humor into the atmosphere but to adjust their mood and conversation to hers. I asked her how long she anticipated needing this intense level of support. "It may take years," she replied, "and if it does, I expect my support system to give me that amount of time."

This type of social authority can become very powerful, even addicting—health never commands such clout. When I asked my new acquaintance what motivation she would have for healing, given her "comfort with her discomfort," so to speak, she was insulted by my question and by my inability to "honor her wounds." Even though I attempted to explain that I was genuinely trying to understand her healing process, she never answered my question.

People also use woundology to make powerful romantic connections. Many people have admitted to me that they come to workshops more for the social contacts than for any actual need to heal. Because loneliness has become so rampant in our culture, when two single, available individuals meet in a workshop, the intimacy of the information they so commonly exchange is often mistaken for romance. There are even "thirteen-steppers"— people who use a twelve-step support group to "hit on" potential romantic partners in vulnerable states of mind.

Many people describe their "soul mate" as the person they have finally found who understands the emotional pain they had experienced as children. Such a bond can certainly feel romantic in the early stages of a relationship, but its foundation is actually injury, pain, and fear. In this paradigm, pain becomes a prerequisite for remaining close to and needing one another, and healing can be seen as a positive threat to the bond. The partnership is inevitably threatened when one of them decides the time has come to release the past and move on.

Don't get me wrong—support groups of all kinds, from AA and other twelve-step programs to those that help people who have lost a parent during childhood, can provide vital assistance and insight. The sharing of wounds has obviously provided a climate that frees people—sometimes for the first time in their lives—to recall their painful memories and explore their feelings and fears with sympathetic, nonjudgmental companions dedicated to supporting them.

The warm and understanding atmosphere that is an almost automatic by-product of this level of sharing also offers group members a social life that may have been missing from their lives prior to joining the group. Another acquaintance of mine, Jane, told me, "The people in my support group, as far as I am concerned, have become my new family. I don't feel judged by them as I do with my biological family. Now I don't feel the need to see my family at all." Certainly the healing intention behind these many support groups is honorable and deserves to be acknowledged; numerous people have benefited and continue to benefit from participating in them.

In addition to all the healing support that they provide, however, another dynamic has made me begin to question their healing value. Those for whom the support group has become an important part of their social life naturally wish to continue indefinitely as members. But because the underlying criterion for remaining a member is a continuing need for support, one must accept the group message "Remain unhealed." That is, to stay a part of the group, you have to "remain apart" from other friends and family.

This dynamic calls to mind a famous saying of the Buddha. "My teachings are a raft," he said, "meant to help you cross over the river. Once you get to the other shore, set them down and go on with your life." "The other shore" was the Buddha's way of describing enlightenment, the goal of his teachings. Once enlightened, continue to live your life, he was saying—just don't carry the raft around with you!

We are not meant to stay wounded. We are supposed to move through our tragedies and challenges and to help each other move through the many painful episodes of our lives. By remaining stuck in the power of our wounds, we block our own transformation. We overlook the greater gifts inherent in our wounds—the strength to overcome them and the lessons that we are meant to receive through them. Wounds are the means through which we enter the hearts of other people. They are meant to teach us to become compassionate and wise.

What would happen, for example, if Jane's support group were to tell her that their role is to give her the strength to heal her unfinished business with her family rather than to become her substitute family? Suppose they told her that as long as she avoided her family with such anger, she was actually running away and not healing, and that she had only a limited amount of time during which the group would help her develop coping skills with her family. At the end of that time, she would be expected to re-enter her biological family, to evaluate her own stamina and strength, to see if she could now interact with them without expecting or needing their approval. If she could do that, she would have healed her major wound.

I actually suggested this to Jane, but she immediately became defensive. To her, leaving her newfound family would be like entering an emotional black hole. So intensely had she bonded with her support group that she could not imagine herself able to cope in her world without them. As far as she was concerned, her group was more than a weekly meeting; it was the center of her social life. She could not think of reaching closure with them, even though they required her to remain "actively wounded" and in need of healing.

YOUR "CELLULAR BANK ACCOUNT"

To understand the dangerous implications of woundology, we first need to look at the nature of the energy that powers our life on earth. Each of us has hundreds of circuits of energy connecting to us, energy that different cultures have named in different ways as the Divine breath of life that animates each of us. What the Indians call *prana* and the Chinese call *ch'i*, Christians refer to as *grace* or *the Holy Spirit*, and secularists might call *vitality* or simply *life-force*. You may think of this energy as flowing into us from the universe, from God, or from the Tao, but as it flows through us, it gives us the juice we need to feed our physical bodies, our minds, and our emotions, as well as to manage our external environments. Everything in our lives—every thought we have, every action we are involved with—requires some of this energy. Although the life-force is equally available to all of us and flows into us whether or not we are aware of it—just as God "makes his sun rise on the evil and on the good, and sends his rain on the just and on the unjust" (Matthew 5:45) —it's possible to maximize our intake and use of it. In fact, consciousness means awareness of the flow of life-force into us and the ability to direct it into certain areas of the body, without unknowingly releasing it from other areas of the body.

Imagine this flow of energy as a financial allowance equal to one hundred dollars per day. Your task is to learn how to invest this money wisely, because your investments will either earn you interest or put you in debt. Obviously, positive investments will earn you positive returns, not only increasing your energy but also creating an energetic surplus. Negative investments, on the other hand, will create debt. If the debt becomes more expensive than your daily allowance, you have to borrow money. In energy terms, you have to borrow energy.

This extra energetic cash is obtainable mainly from two sources. One source is the energy of other people, toward whom you may behave parasitically as a means of supplying your own system. If you use the energy of others in this way, you will eventually become addicted to it and grow more needy and helpless by the day. More and more, you will look to others to boost your self-esteem or to give you ideas of how to live, act, or think, because you no longer have the energy to create your own life. This source of energy is usually short-lived because the people who are your "suppliers" will soon realize that being around you makes them feel that their energy is being drained, and they will avoid you.

The other source of additional energetic cash is the energetic resources held in your own cell tissue. Every cell in your body must have a fresh supply of energy each day in order to thrive, just as they also require fresh water every day. Your daily allowance of one hundred energetic dollars is meant to be used for the everyday maintenance of your physical and emotional life system. Keeping your physical body energized consequently feeds your creativity, your relationships, and your vital need for optimism. But when too much energetic cash is drawn out of your cell bank account, you become debt-ridden. The greater the debt becomes, the weaker your cell tissue grows. If you do not reverse this pattern by paying off our debt with your daily allowance, then you will become vulnerable to the development of disease.

Holding on to the negative events of our histories is expensive—prohibitively so. It is like trying to keep the dead alive, and it takes an enormous amount of energy. When we experience a trauma, Nature supplies us with extra financing, so to speak, to protect us during the draining period of crisis, but that "loan" has a time limit on it. No loan goes on forever, and the signal that the loan is coming due is that we begin to sense that time has come to a standstill, and our lives are not moving forward. When we refuse to let go of pain in our systems, we become depressed. The toxic energy of depression fuels our negative attitudes toward others and drains our own resources further. Soon we project onto others the causes of our own failure and blame them for our bleak condition. This irresponsible response to our problems becomes ordinary and routine. We cling to the negative events and relationships from our past, as well as our present, because they give us permission to see ourselves as victims and everyone else as the source of our misery.

The only way to release the pattern into which we have locked ourselves is to release the weight of the past—to get out of the energy debt we can no longer afford to carry. Forgiveness is one sure way out of debt. Forgiving does not mean saying that what happened to you doesn't matter, or that it is all right for someone to have violated you. It simply means releasing the negative feelings you have about that event and the person or persons involved. This is clearly a difficult and complex psychological process, and I will have much more to say about forgiveness in Chapter 3. But the value of forgiveness is made explicit in the Christian Gospel, where Jesus actually forgives his murderers as he is on the cross, as a prelude to releasing the energy necessary to carry out the Resurrection. And when speaking of prayer, which for Jesus was the key to communion with the Divine, he made it very plain: "Whenever you stand praying, forgive, if you have anything against anyone; so that your Father also who is in heaven will forgive you your offenses" (Mark 11:25). Clearly, Divine energy will not flow into you if you are unwilling to forgive—and move on with your life.

Forgiveness is extraordinarily valuable, but it isn't the only way to free up energy. Some of the events in the past that we need to release are not negative events but good times. You may not be able to let go of the fact that you are no longer twenty—you are fifty, or eighty. You may not be able to let go of the youthful appearance you once had, or your athletic ability, or the quickness of your mind. This inability is another way of losing energy by spending it on the past. One of my dearest friends could not let go of her college years. At that time in her life, she had felt that the entire world was awaiting her and that she could do anything. But after college, each time some opportunity came up, she would find a reason not to take advantage of it. In fact, she was afraid that she didn't really want to do anything. The combination of her fear of engaging life and clinging to a moment in the past that seemed filled with potential finally bankrupted her energetic account, and a terminal disease was manifested. Twenty years after the fact, she was still obsessed with her college years and could not get on with her life. A few years ago, she developed lupus and died—lupus being tied directly to fear of letting go.

In a similar way, many women in their fifties and sixties hold on to their thirties by wearing youthful styles when they should be acknowledging that they are at the wisdom, or mentoring, or crone stage of their lives. Aging men do the same thing by buying a red sports car and chasing women in their twenties. These are all toxic behaviors and can be just as deleterious to health as refusing to let go of negative events from the past. You have to accept the stage of life in which you find yourself and maintain it with consciousness. If you're in your later years, you need not accept that this stage of life means decay, but you can't live in regret that your early years are gone.

Refusing to let go of past events, whether positive or negative, means throwing away some part of your daily energy budget. If you start losing energy and don't do anything about it, you will inevitably develop a weakness in your physical body. The problem may begin simply enough, when you begin to feel "off" or notice that your energy level is low. If you don't pay attention, that may lead to developing a viral infection, flu, headache, migraine, or nausea. If you continue to lose energy without taking action, those minor upsets can develop into major illnesses. And although it's an unpopular idea, susceptibility to accidents, I think, can be part of the scenario. An "accident-prone" person is actually energetically in debt. He or she is out of balance and is susceptible to everything from minor clumsiness to a life-threatening accident. Such people have to learn to recognize these days or stretches of time—just as we may "feel a cold coming on" and try to get extra rest or take supplements—because that's not the time to go for a job interview or make major decisions.

As a medical intuitive, I happen to see more easily than others the precise workings of energy loss—although, as I showed in *Anatomy of the Spirit*, you can learn to diagnose yourself with a little practice. The diagnostic readings I do involve following the energy circuits I see going into a person and "reading" what they tell me. Following a circuit is a little like reading an EKG—you look for blips indicating danger. I go backward in time, and when I come to a blip in the circuit, I wait for impressions about what happened, which begin to tell me where the person has left some of his spirit.

Some years ago I did one reading on a woman with chronic pain. When I had gone back eleven years into her past, I sensed that she had lost her daughter in a car accident. That is a very legitimate injury and wound; in fact, our society would probably put that wound on sacred ground as perhaps the highest of all social wounds.

As I observed her energy circuit, the wound changed in its image to a life raft with too many passengers in it. I watched it for a while longer, and suddenly I realized that I was dealing with an extremely manipulative woman who, for the first time in her life, had received a legitimate wound and by no means was going to let go of it. Did she grieve the loss of her daughter? Yes, of course. But another part of her personality thought, "This ain't bad." She used the wound to legitimize her manipulative self. I often see people do this: They take a legitimate grievance from a hard childhood and convert it to the right to be manipulative, bitter, or angry. This woman later acknowledged that she was an extremely unethical person in her business, and that anytime somebody challenged her, she would pull out her wound. They would end up apologizing to her: "Oh my God, I'm so sorry I challenged you." Ask yourself: Who is going to give up that kind of power?

So I said to her, in effect, "I realize that the loss of your daughter was very serious and very intense, and I'm not questioning that. But you have made the best of a very bad situation, and the best of it is that you are getting mileage out of this wound that makes the release of it absolutely impossible. This wound has given you a level of clout that you never had before." She acknowledged that it was so. I could see in her face, even as she did so, how much she still wanted to hold on to that wound.

Why is it so hard to give up a wound? I believe that we are all born with a certain packet of perceptions, of "that which we know to be true." One of the perceptions in that packet is that if we let go of certain things, our lives are going to change. And the reality is that we are actually more afraid of change than we are of death. I once gave a lecture on this subject at the University of New Hampshire, to an audience of maybe six hundred people. One woman, who otherwise had a very quiet, even meek demeanor, tentatively asked me to clarify what I was saying about giving up our language of woundology. I answered that we don't want to give it up because it's become our first language of intimacy, and we've created everything else—our romantic life, our social life— around bonding with wounds. To most people, I said, the idea of giving that up is too shattering. At this point the woman suddenly shot out of her seat as if an electrical charge had just gone through her chair. "I don't like what you're saying," she shouted. "I do not like it, because if I gave up this language of wounds, I would have nothing to say to anybody. I don't like this one bit!"

THE SOCIAL WOUND

Cases like this woman's and Jane's are not rare. Woundology has become a widespread social phenomenon, representing a shift in global consciousness. During the past four decades

American society has made a substantial effort to become sensitized to the need for people to heal from personal trauma, losses, and violations. Our culture has become more aware of post-traumatic stress disorders, as well as the impact of emotional and sexual violations that prior to the 1960s were virtually invisible. The sexual revolution, the holistic health movement, and the therapeutic culture opened the tribal mind to recognizing the criminal magnitude of these kinds of personal violations, which it had previously viewed less as traumatic than as physical injuries.

Once the Tribal mind—the most primitive, survival-oriented level of social consciousness, identified with ethnicity, nationality, and consensus reality—recognized the psychological and emotional consequences of these violations, it responded by forming support groups for the emotionally injured and bypassing laws that criminalized psychological and emotional violations. These and other healing measures were appropriate and much needed.

But probably because emotional wounds are so powerful, cultural attitudes have now extended beyond appropriate healing measures to become hypersensitive to the claims and demands of victims. Teachers, physicians, clergy, businesspeople, and even family members must suddenly exercise extreme caution in dealing with children or members of the opposite sex, lest they risk allegations of "inappropriate" behavior.

On my own workshop circuit, a contract I received contained an advisory on a "new policy on harassment" identifying nine categories of behavioral patterns that are now officially recognized as offensive (read: wound-causing). These behavior patterns are "subtle and not-so-subtle ranging from joke telling to touching to offensive verbal conduct to failing to take action in reporting the offensive behavior of another person."

Obviously, people who were abused and tormented during their youth often need help in facing their histories and evaluating their actions. Yet adults who suffered childhood abuse do have alternatives to murdering their abusers. Policies such as these, although well-meaning, encourage people to "seek out the wound" in social settings and to look for offensive behavior in what could actually be completely innocent circumstances. An Episcopal priest recently told me of her deep distress regarding the new policy of her church, which forbids hugging or embracing of any parishioner. "As a spiritual director, I often touch clients in a supportive way," she said. "I am now not allowed to touch anyone and have to leave the door open during sessions of spiritual direction or confession, which are totally private." Her response to the policy was to get certification as a massage therapist and bodyworker so that she would have, as it were, license to touch.

The power of the wound has become potent in our courts as well, as the hung jury in the initial 1995 trial of the Menendez brothers showed. In our efforts to create a society that is more conscious of the feelings of its members, we must now ask ourselves if we have gone too far in encouraging people to be mindful of one another's wounds. Attorneys now routinely advertise on television, encouraging people to sue others for "personal injury," which amounts to earning money by staying wounded and angry. The social message is that wounds are a means to profit; healing earns you nothing. Woundology finally amounts to a kind of welfare state of the soul, paying people dividends for blithely refusing to better their condition.

In our fast-paced information culture, the rules that govern our lives are changing almost faster than we can comprehend. The cultural response to the new awareness of emotional wounds has been to become wound-sensitized, because all healing—be it for an individual or for an entire society—begins with the identification of wounds. But identification of wounds is only the first stage of healing: The actual journey of healing requires moving through that pain.

I'm not suggesting that as individuals we ignore the effects of our wounds on our day-to-day behavior. But we must also avoid dwelling on past traumas, to the point of depleting the energy available for running our bodies, and diverting energy from the present for whatever reason. The whole point of "consciousness," as we use that term, is to learn to *be conscious* of precisely these kinds of subtle energetic developments in the body and spirit, and to act accordingly.

Developing this consciousness has extremely wide-ranging implications for how we live. An actual vibrational or energy exchange that happens when we're outdoors, for example, is different from one that happens when we're indoors, or when we're in sunlight as opposed to when we're away from sunlight. When we're outdoors, it's not just that we feel warm in the sun and get a suntan; a vibrational field actually merges with our own and enhances the quality or the flow of energy through our body. To put it in plain terms, the effect of sunlight on our energy system is similar to that of a battery being charged. Developing consciousness involves learning the behaviors that charge our energy cells and keep us vital.

Conversely, when we neglect or abuse energy and life, we pay an energetic debt for that. Viewing a trauma or a tragedy happening in somebody else's life demands of us a compassionate response, since compassion is an energy charge that assists a suffering person. If we respond without compassion, however, or dismiss the whole event, we may incur a karmic debt. As we begin to learn how powerful energy is—that it is absolutely the core of life, not just a measurement of vigor—we will discover the power contained in our thoughts, as applied not just to ourselves but to other people.

One of the most profound stories that I ever heard in a workshop was told by a woman who had been seriously injured in a car accident and had had a near-death experience—I'll call her Maggie. Maggie was so shattered that she went out of her body, and in that state, floating above the scene of the accident, she could hear how people in cars behind her were responding to the accident. Some were deeply shaken by witnessing it, while others were saying things like "Oh, Jesus, this is all I need! How long are we going to be stuck here?" But from the fifth car behind hers, she saw a beautiful swirl of light rising up into the ether and then right back down into her own body. She thought, "What's going on there?" And just as she thought that, she was instantly next to the woman in that car, who was sending out a prayer for her. In that energetic state, in the midst of her near-death experience, Maggie got the license plate of that car and committed it to memory. She eventually came back into her body and was taken to the hospital. When she was fully recovered, she tracked down the woman who had prayed for her, and she showed up at her doorstep with a bouquet of flowers to say thank you.

SPIRIT RETRIEVAL

In tracking the souls of some people with cancer, I have often seen that early in their lives, a figure of some significance—a parent or teacher perhaps—said something to them like "You'll never be good enough" or "You'll never amount to anything." It may have taken only three seconds, yet those three seconds commanded the rest of the person's life. If you can be totally commanded by a three-second comment, do you really think you create your own reality? I don't think so. It is that negativity that is creating your reality, and your challenge is to become strong enough to call your spirit back.

As you read the next few pages and perform the following exercise, keep in mind that you really do create your own reality. Imagine a big circle in front of you, and then visualize your *prana*, your life-force or grace, coming into the top of your head. Now you're given the choice: How do you want to distribute your prana? As you distribute it, so it will come back to you—what goes around, comes around. You say to your spirit, "Go back to this bitter event in my past and keep it alive for me, and then bring me the harvest from it." And from that harvest you feed your cell tissue.

Exercise: Calling Your Spirit Back

By no means is it easy to retrieve your spirit from days gone by, not only because genuine hurt is involved, but also because dwelling on sad or anger-filled memories can become a habit—almost like being under a spell. We become accustomed to dwelling in yesterday's junk mail simply because we are used to it. So easily does our spirit go to our historic burial grounds that its energy bypasses our conscious mind and then simply alerts us that it has taken its position in our past. Thus, over time, we no longer even have to consciously activate our unhappy past; it is activated automatically.

The process of retrieving this energy from the past begins by making a shift in awareness and vocabulary; simply put, you have to outrun your past. Learn to become conscious, as often as possible, of what you are thinking about and where your energy is. When you feel yourself drifting back into the fog of a memory, command your energy to return to the present moment by saying, "I am not going in that direction any longer. I release it once and for all." And don't make heavy weather out of the act of releasing. It isn't always necessary to beat up pillows on the floor while screaming in rage. Release can also be accomplished with a bit of humor, such as, "You again? Beat it! I haven't got either the time or the energy to think about you any longer." Lighten up, and don't allow your past to frighten you. Stop giving it power by clinging to the belief that things could or should have been otherwise. That is nonsense.

As you gain more control over your thoughts, try changing your vocabulary too. Speak more in the present tense about your life. You can certainly recall your past, but make it a habit to recall the good times. When someone asks you how you are, give them a positive answer; let that be your default setting. If you are genuinely coping with something that recently happened to you, go ahead and share that, but don't dwell on it. If the incident reminds you of the "many other times this has happened to me," then recall those times *if and only if* you are finally prepared to try to understand and break the pattern within you that is somehow involved in their creation. If, in your sojourn into your past memories, you emerge feeling even more like a victim, saying, "See? I just can't win, no matter what I do," then you are missing the point of calling your spirit back. To heal the past you have to "time travel" with the genuine intention of seeking and breaking repetitious patterns and gaining insights into what you need to learn in this lifetime.

✦

Chapter Two

THE FIVE MYTHS
ABOUT HEALING

The connection between consciousness and illness is currently the object of much speculation and scientific research. Certainly, becoming conscious of negative beliefs and their effects on us can help us make positive choices and change our lives for the better. I believe, along with many other teachers and researchers, that an awareness of the innate connection between our body-mind and our spirit can catalyze a healing.

Nonetheless, even the holiest of people can and do become ill. Extraordinarily saintly people have contracted the commonest diseases, including painful cancers. Some may even have known in advance how they would die. Yet despite their physical challenges, these saints and sages still strove to understand themselves, to exercise compassion toward others, and to connect with the Divine energy that directed their lives. While they may not have cured themselves of physical illness—or even tried to do so—they healed into an acceptance of Divine will and the higher purpose for their lives.

We need to realize that in some cases it may be Divine will that we do not heal at the physical level but learn from a chronic or terminal disease certain lessons that our soul needs to discover. At other times, we are meant to absorb spiritual virtues that are available to us only through illness and perhaps by doing so, inspire others. Transformation through illness is a time-honored spiritual theme, and faith in the Divine can yield dramatic insight and healing.

In carrying his cross on the way to his crucifixion, Jesus was helped for a while by a man named Simon. That symbolically powerful incident is deserving of far more attention than it has been given: It is saying that in our journey toward selfhood and toward realizing our unique destinies, we have to also carry burdens for those who aren't strong enough—and sometimes the burden is negativity.

Once when I was in London, I did a reading on an exquisite man who had the face of someone who is blessed. He came up to me after my lecture and said, "I'm a very good person, but I don't understand why I have so much difficulty with the authorities where I work." He worked for British Telecom. I looked at him and saw nothing but kindness coming out of his auric field. I closed my eyes and asked for guidance, and I got a very strong impression that he was a kind of guardian angel in training and was absorbing a lot of negativity. Much of the negativity was racist, because he was from India. A lot of other Indians he knew were also experiencing that racism but were not strong enough to deal with it, so he absorbed the blows for them. I explained this to the man, adding, "I don't know if this is going to help you, but it is the only impression I have."

"Oh," he said, "I could live with that." I heard an even more surprising story about a highly respected Indian teacher who developed terminal multiorgan cancer. He became weaker as his illness progressed, and his body began to show outward signs of the inner ravaging. One day a devoted student approached him and inquired why he wasn't healing himself—or couldn't heal himself. The spiritual master turned to him and laughed. "You want to see me heal this?" he said. "Watch." And with that, the master healed his body, which instantly resumed its former healthy glow—causing his student even more confusion.

"I don't understand," said the student. "If you have so much light in you, what then is causing this darkness of disease?"

"This isn't my darkness," replied the spiritual master. "It is yours and my other students'. I am carrying it for you until you are strong enough to carry it for yourself. As for me, I feel none of it."

Accepting Divine direction is the key to growing in spiritual maturity—and it is also the key to healing both physical and emotional challenges. Regardless of whether an illness is a spiritual crisis or has developed from negativity, human nature is designed to seek a means of healing. Yet my many experiences in working with people confronting illness have caused me to believe that people often do not heal because, either consciously or unconsciously, they have more faith in deeply potent belief patterns that interfere with healing than they do in their ability to heal.

There are five central myths about healing that can fully take charge of a person's mental and emotional strength and make healing nearly impossible. Each of them supports the consciousness of woundology, which serves to weaken the body far more than to repair it. These belief patterns are so powerful that they sometimes seem to be stronger than our optimistic beliefs about the possibility of healing. This is because hopeful, optimistic beliefs are about the future, about possibilities, whereas illness is a reality and the myths that support it are in the present time. Healing is intangible, but you can feel and see your illness.

The most effective way to break the controlling force of a myth is to recognize that you personally believe it, and that while you may share this belief with others, it is a belief and not necessarily a fact. Then work consciously to detach yourself from its influence. As you read about each of the five myths, ask yourself: "Is this something I believe?" If you find that you do, I will provide ways—through prayers and other rituals—to loosen their grip on your mind. No myth releases itself from the psyche without a fight, yet if you are intent on genuine healing, you have no choice but to carry on that fight and then develop thought-forms to supplant them and support your health.

THE FIRST MYTH:
MY LIFE IS DEFINED BY MY WOUND

It is virtually impossible not to be influenced by a personal history of emotional or psychological wounds. Both literally and symbolically, wounds permeate our blood and bodies. Our biographies are in large part biologies. Wounds are like diversionary canals that drain water and spirit out of the river of our life. The more wounds we have, the more effort we have to put into calling our energy back, stopping up the energy drains, and otherwise attending to our healing process. No matter the number and depth of those diversions, healing requires that our life-force be redirected back into our own life.

Many people come to believe, however, that their lives are only a compilation of psychological wounds, which they feel they can do little to heal. To the suggestion that their wounds can be released, such people often respond, "You don't understand. I have never been the same since that experience. How can I change that now?"

After experiencing a traumatic or tragic experience, these people tend to look at every new experience through the lens of the wound it inflicted on them. They project their past experience onto everything that has since come into their lives. They enter every new relationship suspecting that the same pattern of the experience will repeat itself. They warn every new person who enters their life that they will never be able to trust him or her fully because of their previous experience. And they describe their life as a continuum of personal and professional disasters that cannot change because their wounded past has stolen from them all positive opportunities that could have or should have come their way.

Although this state of mind is sad, self-limiting, and defeatist, some people derive great power in maintaining it because it gives permission to lead a life of minimum expectation and limited responsibility. It allows them to lean on others for assistance and to play on their guilt to keep that assistance coming. They speak regretfully or bitterly about creative goals that they cannot accomplish, now or ever, because of their history of emotional or physical abuse. They seek out a support system that gives them a social comfort zone, one that will remain sympathetic to their woundedness without ever challenging them to put it behind them. Since nothing is expected of the wounded personality, they can never fail.

As the years go by, as these people become accustomed to this kind of power and self-protection, they find it more and more difficult to change. The older we get, the harder it is to step out of our wounds and into a different view of life. Yet the fact is that emphasizing your wounds can damage your psyche as much as the original wounds did. Dwelling on a wound is, in fact, a type of self-inflicted wound, a self-flagellation, in which your consciousness is always focused on weakness and never on recovery. Further, a psyche that believes in its own emotional and psychological vulnerability can only produce a physical body that reflects the same "full house," as they say in poker. If you fear strength and independence, you will find it very difficult to retain or recover your health.

In one workshop I encountered a man named Frank who was deeply entrenched in the belief that his wounds had created an inalterable limitation on what he could accomplish in his life. Frank continually commented that he could have become a scientist or a physician, but because some of his grade school teachers had constantly criticized him, he had no alternative but to choose jobs that required less education so that he could avoid further humiliation.

During the course of the workshop, whenever the discussion turned to the effects of various medical treatment, Frank immediately added his opinion, which was always negative. Physicians don't really know what they are doing when it comes to treating illness, he said, because most of them have no personal experience of what it's like to suffer severely. At one point in the workshop, another man objected that many physicians come from difficult personal backgrounds, and that they have chosen the medical profession as a way of helping others. He himself was such a physician, he said. Frank dismissed this objection, suggesting that the physician was merely repressing his pain and that as a doctor he could not get in touch with his emotions. As the discussion progressed through the afternoon, four people spoke of their success at healing their personal histories. But Frank clearly found their positive comments threatening. He finally stood up and announced that no one had been as emotionally injured as he had—and he left the group!

In spite of Frank's attitude, I was deeply inspired by the wonderful healing stories that others in this group shared, as I have been by the many I have heard in other workshops. People have pulled themselves through nightmarish experiences and gone on to build not only productive lives but also joyful ones.

In one workshop a woman named Alison shared her experience of healing breast cancer. Shortly after she turned thirty, she discovered a lump in her breast, which proved to be malignant. At the time of the diagnosis, Alison was involved with Sam, and they were beginning to talk about getting married. When she told him of her condition, he said that together they "would fight this thing" and then get on with their lives. It didn't turn out that way, however, because as Alison put it, "he needed me to depend on him. Dependency made him feel secure in the relationship because it gave him a feeling of control."

As Alison worked on healing her body, she also healed her personality enough to realize that although she loved Sam, her dependence on him was blocking her progress. So strong was her dependence on him, in fact, that she was actually looking to him to do the healing for her. At the same time, she feared becoming strong herself because she associated strength with independence. "I had no idea how to relate to anyone without giving them a list of my vulnerable points," she said. "I knew how to be incomplete, which always seemed to be a means of getting close to someone. I mean, it sure worked with Sam and the other men I had been involved with. But now I had to become a whole different kind of person, someone who was strong and able to face cancer alone."

Even the thought of healing something by herself was frightening to Alison, because it might give Sam the impression that she was doing something that didn't require him the way she always had in the past. "I was actually as tormented by my fear of being healed as I was of not healing," she said. "I realized that being a healed person meant that I would have to challenge all those parts of myself that had always been my way of communicating with people, especially Sam. I decided one evening that I had to make a choice, and so I told Sam that I needed 'some space' to pull myself together. He took this to mean that I was rejecting him; that was more or less the end of our relationship."

Alison's physician finally gave her a different perspective. Being a stronger person did not mean living alone, she told Alison, but rather living a better life, because independence means choice. Strength would put her in a position where she did not have to "settle for what came along" but could make choices as to whom she wanted to be with. "I didn't believe her at first, but I sure liked what she was saying," Alison said.

Alison recalled those words every time she slipped into her fears of aloneness—particularly now that she was actually living alone. "I got to the point where I told myself that alone or with someone, I wanted to live a good and healthy life," she said. "And the thing I find so interesting about that decision is that once I said that to myself, I started to believe that I could handle my life alone. Yet at the same time that I knew I would not be alone."

After our conversation I felt very positive about Alison's condition. I saw in her all of the elements of commitment and backbone that a person needs when facing a serious illness. But more than that, I saw she knew that to be the truth. I later received a letter from Allison telling me that her cancer had gone into remission and that she was fully confident that she would accomplish a full healing.

I do not underestimate the difficulty of letting go of the belief that your life is and always will be defined by your wounds. This myth is particularly difficult to give up because it is so serviceable: It allows us to feel that any failure or absence of accomplishment on our part is someone else's fault. The only way to release the grip this myth has on your psyche is to take more responsibility for the quality of your life, as Alison did. Instead of stating that you wish you had gone to college, go to college. Start by taking one course at a time, by correspondence if necessary, but start. Instead of wishing you weighed fifty pounds less than you do, start walking and change your diet, even if you walk just one mile a day and eliminate only a few high-fat foods. When you find yourself saying or thinking, "I could have been a ———, but my wounded past prevented me from achieving it," then take steps to fulfill precisely that "impossible" goal.

Questions for Self-Examination

+ Do you make excuses for why you're not doing more positive things with your life?

+ Do you compare your history of wounds with others? If so, why?

+ If you feel more wounded than someone else, does that make you feel more empowered?

THE SECOND MYTH:
BEING HEALTHY MEANS BEING ALONE

A phrase commonly used to refer to a return to health is "to stand on one's own two feet again"—that is, to take care of oneself, to be independent. But to some psychologically wounded people, becoming healthy and attaining independence would amount to isolation and vulnerability. For many, this fear of heroic independence—and by extension, of being alone—lies at the core of their inability to heal. Moreover, they believe, once they are healed, they will always be healed, and so with the onset of health the need for emotional and psychological support will somehow evaporate altogether. This is another variant of the archaic belief that once we reach the Promised Land, we have no more traveling to do. But people who are healing and who are healed need companionship and friendship like anyone else. We create health every day and all the time, and we need to do so consciously. Just as enlightenment is not a one-time event achievable only by spiritual supermen, health doesn't occur outside of a community—it requires a conscious connection between mind, body, and spirit, a connection between the individual, other people, and the greater universe.

Healing, like spirituality, is an ongoing process, as many insightful stories from the Eastern tradition make clear. In one story related by Insight Meditation teacher and psychologist Jack Kornfield, a Zen monk walks up a mountain determined to find enlightenment or die. On the way up, he meets a wise old man carrying a big bundle and asks him if he knows about enlightenment. The old man, who is actually the Bodhisattva of Wisdom, drops the bundle on the ground. The monk immediately becomes enlightened.

"You mean it's that simple?" he says. "Just let go and don't grasp anything!" Then he looks at the old man and asks, "What now?"

The old man reaches down, picks up the bundle again, and walks off to the village. That is, even after enlightenment, the same pleasures and tasks await us. Even after healing, we have to keep working on our healing. Healing is not a process that has an ending.

In American society the prevailing attitude is that a healthy person is one who has recovered completely from a past injury or illness and is able to go on with his or her life immune to any further health problems. Yet the truth is that whether we are healed or are in the process of healing, we will always need a community of loving friends and family—a community based not solely on wounds or neediness but also on shared interests and emotional nurturing. Healing does not represent the closure of the needs of the heart; rather, it is a doorway toward opening your heart.

America has long been in love with the myth of the rugged individualist. The problem is that very few of us can fully identify with that icon because we are essentially social beings. As long as we believe that genuine healing requires a heroic individual effort, we will have a convenient excuse not to begin to try. Often undertaking even modest healing measures, like learning meditation and yoga or changing our diets, will seem insurmountable if we can't envision doing them with at least one willing partner, though certainly many have pursued these changes by themselves.

At one of my workshops, a woman named Beth told me that being diagnosed with cancer motivated her to seek healing through complementary medicine. She changed her diet and stopped smoking and drinking alcohol. Then she joined a cancer support group, turned to a therapist for assistance, and began to practice yoga. Her boyfriend Matt, who was a heavy smoker, found these efforts enormously threatening, especially when she told him that he could no longer smoke in their home.

Beth and Matt started to battle continually, both about smoking and about the time she was now spending away from home. Feeling he had less and less in common with Beth, Matt demanded that she move out of their house. She admitted to me that this was the one change she had feared the most, not only because she lacked the financial resources to find a new residence and meet her medical expenses, but also because she had been involved with Matt for so long that she could not imagine life without him.

Beth suggested a compromise: Matt could smoke in the house and eat whatever he wanted, and she would limit going to her support group to every other week. In return, he would no longer criticize her for keeping to her new diet or for attending her yoga class.

When I asked Beth if this new plan was working out, she replied, "Well, I'm doing most of what I should be doing, so I have that on my side. But I miss the weekly support group meetings, because Matt can't really relate to what it's like to have cancer. Those people can, and I feel accepted by them. We share a mutual goal, and we care about each other. I like that feeling; in fact, I love that feeling. Matt says they're not all that interested in me, only in getting what they can from me for their own benefit. I don't really believe that, but I can't prove it to him because he refuses to meet the group. At any rate, he did promise that he'd stick it out with me, and I guess that's what really matters the most."

I don't know whether Beth eventually healed her illness, but I hope that she came to see how her energy was being compromised by her dilemma. However, when I think of her, I see a person whose focus was not actually on healing, but on not being alone, and that the fear "aloneness" held for her would more likely fuel her illness rather than her effort to recover her health.

On another occasion I met a sparkling young man named Bart who had been diagnosed with leukemia. Within two days of his diagnosis, he had plunged into reading everything he could get his hands on that related to mind-body healing methods. He changed every part of his life, including repainting his apartment with colors that he felt encouraged tranquillity.

Only one of Bart's friends actually showed any respect for what he was doing. The others teased him, especially when he began to eat only organic food and started a spiritual practice. He eventually cut off contact with his old circle of friends, and although he missed them at first, he remained focused totally on recovering his health. He was willing to live in a world of complete isolation and silence if that was what he had to do to heal.

Bart's new lifestyle was indeed somewhat isolating. Yet isolation became a soothing companion for him. In fact, he started to like and respect the person he was becoming. He enjoyed feeling strong and confident about his newfound ability to handle his life, even though at times he missed socializing with his old friends. But no matter how lonely he felt, he comforted himself by visualizing his future with positive images of a new life, not of loneliness but of hope, surrounded by friends. Within two years, he was fully in remission. I later heard from someone close to Bart that he had married and made new friends who shared his love of organic food and spiritual practice.

The requirements for healing are tough ones, especially if they demand that we let go of some or all of our intimate companions. While letting go is certainly not necessary for everyone to do, when it is necessary, it is the only real choice to make. If you need to let go of old friends, keep in mind the cyclical nature of life, extolled by mystics from the unknown author of Ecclesiastes to Lao-tzu. After winter comes spring. Loneliness and friendship can each play a role on your healing at different times—or even at different moments within the same time period. Healing doesn't require isolation, any more than mysticism requires hair shirts and a diet of locusts.

Questions for Self-Examination

+ Are you afraid that if you heal, your support group will abandon you or be less sympathetic to you?

+ When you picture yourself as healed, are you the only one in the room?

+ Do you see emotional wounds as a means of bonding with another person, and does healing mean having to separate from that person?

THE THIRD MYTH: FEELING PAIN
MEANS BEING DESTROYED BY PAIN

It is often the case that pain represents the presence of illness, either emotional or physical, and it is normal to believe that all pain is negative. But pain is also a teacher, a messenger directing us to pay attention to our bodies or to move away from behavior and situations in which we are weak to those in which we practice integrity and strength.

Our drug-filled society maintains that most physically and psychologically painful conditions should be medicated away. Television commercials support the use of painkilling remedies for headaches, backaches, and every other symptom imaginable. Undeniably, chronic pain is a serious handicap to living a full life, and it makes maintaining a positive attitude enormously difficult. Yet emotional and psychological pain can also be a signal to pay attention. It can be a teacher, whether it originates in our emotions or our physical bodies. It directs our attention to the physical or emotional area that is begging for repair. Drugging pain prematurely or too much can be a mistake, because it can mislead us into thinking that we are healing when we are not. Instead of immediately medicating ourselves in every instance, we should examine why we have a pain or a pattern of physical aches and pains. My favorite commercials to dislike are the ones that advertise remedies for upset stomach that you take *before* you eat, so that you can eat all the greasy, spicy, or milk-based food you want while silencing the pain in your stomach that is trying to tell you that your body cannot digest this kind of food.

Although the use of pain-relieving drugs may be essential at some stage in any healing process, we need to ask if those drugs are always necessary or if they have become a distraction from what the pain is telling us about our lives. Being in pain is a horrific experience, but so is drug dependence. Drugs make things worse because when you take them, you cannot feel what is taking place in your body and you may come to believe that the absence of pain is the same as healing. It is not. Do not be afraid of entering pain and using it as an ally to help you repair your body. It may well be that it is the only language that can command your full attention.

If you recognize that a dependence has developed, then consider a gradual program of withdrawal and a support system that can help you with this most difficult task. Before you begin withdrawal from any kind of drug, however, I recommend that you make contact with a therapist who can hold your hand—and your mind, so to speak—and guide you one step at a time into yourself. Learn alternative methods of mind-body control, such as using your breath as a means of communicating with your body, or biofeedback, which was developed for exactly this purpose.

If you are ready to turn your attention to entering your pain, you will probably need help—chances are you won't know where or how to begin. One way to begin is by studying yourself. Pay attention to how many thoughts and attitudes you hold in yourself each day that are painful. Write them down so that you see them in physical form, and recognize the physical damage they can do to your body. You may come to realize that you dwell on painful images of yourself or on pain-filled beliefs about life. You may even realize that you are, at your core, a pessimist, always viewing everything negatively and discounting the positive. Or you may come to recognize that it is not your pain that you are carrying, but the grief of others that you want to protect. It may even become possible for you to understand pain as a spiritual challenge that has come into your life as a means of making your state of mind stronger than you could have imagined possible.

A man named Fred, who came to one of my workshops, revealed that he had started to take painkillers when his back gave him trouble. Although his medication initially brought him relief, he found that as time went on he needed more and more of it. After about a year he told his physician that the medication was no longer effective and asked for a stronger prescription. His physician instead recommended that he do exercises to strengthen his back. He started to follow his advice, but the exercises simply were not working. He then went to a different physician who did give him a stronger medication, but in time even that prescription was "not enough."

When I asked Fred why he hadn't taken a look at the reason his back was in such bad shape, he said, "Quite frankly, I didn't want to be bothered with all that, because it would take too much time and I wanted immediate relief." I asked him what, aside from his back and drug dilemma, was also causing him stress in his life. He said that he had a history of bad financial investments and business deals and that he was always in search of fast and easy ways to make a lot of money. He had even been involved in a pyramid scheme. The more he failed, the more his back ached.

I asked him why he had failed to see the connection between his financial stress and his back problem. He said that he knew these two problems were related, but he told himself that once he made his fortune, his back would heal. He still believed that and was determined to create financial abundance for himself.

When I asked him why he would attend one of my workshops, given his attitude, Fred said that he wanted to learn how to use "mind power" and intuition to help him make better business decisions. I suggested that his painkillers might be interfering with his judgment, but he insisted that the only way he could make any good choices was to be pain-free. We ended the conversation on that note. I did not have high hopes for his recovery.

On the positive side, Lester had experienced tremendous pain from a tumor in his leg and the subsequent surgery to remove the cancerous tissue. During his recovery period he was given pain medication, which he said he needed because the pain was beyond his capacity to cope. During his effort to regain strength in his leg, his pain increased, and it persisted even when he wasn't walking or stretching his leg.

Lester continued on his medication because the throbbing in his leg kept him awake at night, no matter how exhausted he was. One night, as he was lying in bed wondering if he would ever recover from cancer and pain, it occurred to him to focus his attention on entering his pain. He imagined himself traveling into his leg to see what was actually taking place underneath his skin.

He put on some background music to help him relax and pictured himself repairing the cell tissue in his leg and communicating the message that all the cancer cells were to be destroyed immediately. With each passing day that he repeated this practice, his confidence grew, and he began to withdraw gradually from his painkillers. Finally he discontinued them altogether, even though his body was still in some pain. He said that he had begun to look at his pain as a "guiding light" that, with each meditation, told him where to focus his attention.

"Through this daily practice, or I should say hourly practice," Lester concluded, "I actually came to believe, and not just hope, that I could heal my body. I felt my mind get stronger every single day, and I literally felt my body repairing itself."

I had no doubt that Lester was going to make it, and neither did he.

Questions for Self-Examination

+ Do you think of pain as always being an enemy?

+ Have you ever learned anything from physical pain? If so, what?

+ To cope with pain, are you more inclined to take chemical medication or to use meditation or some other inner discipline?

+ Have you ever been addicted to pain medication or sleeping pills?

THE FOURTH MYTH: ALL ILLNESS IS THE RESULT OF NEGATIVITY, AND WE ARE DAMAGED AT OUR CORE

Our thoughts powerfully influence the health of our minds and bodies, and delving into our inner selves is essential to the healing process. Yet negative patterns are not always at the root of illness, and a failure to heal should not always be blamed on negative past experiences or on negative beliefs buried deep in the unconscious mind. Too many people have told me that they have searched long and hard in their background for that missing negative experience, only to come up empty. Why and how, they wonder, can they unearth that missing piece of their psyche?

Sometimes illness is the result of a complex of causes and it can be futile to try to fix the cause on a single, simple factor. Life is just not that simple. Some illnesses develop, for example, because of our increasingly toxic environment as well as exposures to germs, bacteria, and viruses. Others are the result of exposure to contaminated water or parasites. Still others are the result of genetics that may just be impossible to outrun. And some, as stated earlier, can be a form of spiritual guidance. In our quest to become physically and spiritually strong, we have forgotten that our emotional journey is relatively new and that our physical bodies are still subject to powerful dominance by our environments and by the rapidly changing, unsettling patterns in our society.

Healing from illness would be better served if we investigated our past for positive patterns as well as negative ones. Even as we seek out all that can contribute to our weaknesses, we need to bring into focus the strong and enduring parts of our personalities. When people focus only on their negative patterns, all that is good about them and their lives can be eclipsed.

A strong and focused willpower, which is essential to repairing physical tissue, is a rare quality. We tend to use our willpower far more to try to control others than to learn to control ourselves. And when we try to develop a stronger sense of inner will, we are more likely to be motivated by a desire to break an addiction pattern or develop a daily exercise routine than by a wish to control our negative thoughts.

Support programs should not only help people recover from their wounds but also celebrate their strengths. The human spirit does not go to sleep within us because of negative life patterns, nor are most people's lives only a series of tragedies. Unearthing the positive is as effective a healing process as is clearing out the negative parts of our history.

After Sheila was diagnosed with breast cancer, she immediately sought medical care and joined a support group for women with the same illness. As she met with this group, she initially found their sympathy a great help for releasing her grief about her recent divorce, a divorce that she had not wanted. Her desire to find a way to reconnect with her former husband had been, as she put it, "draining the life out of" her, symbolically as well as physically.

Although the support group helped Sheila move through her despair, her cancer was nonetheless progressing. Several members of her group insisted that she must still be holding on to her marriage, or to some other negative part of her past. She could not figure out what it might be, so she came to my workshop to find a way to get in touch with whatever negative emotions she was holding on to.

Until Sheila's marriage began to fall apart, her life had been fairly happy. "Oh sure, I had problems with my kids and a few other things," she admitted, "but all of these problems worked out. My children are now adults, and we have loving relationships with each other. I have never had any financial stress, and though both my parents have died, I believe that it was their time. I mourned their parting, and after a while I was fine."

As Sheila continued to describe her history, I asked her how she felt about herself. I expected her to go into a list of symptoms of low self-esteem, but she surprised me. She said that she had always thought of herself as kind, compassionate, intelligent, and socially comfortable. "Now," she commented, "I'm wondering if I was just kidding myself. Maybe I've never been all those things."

Her self-esteem was absolutely beautiful—and refreshing to see. Yet as I continued talking with her, I began to feel that she was disintegrating right before my eyes. It turned out that she no longer felt so good about herself and recently had become convinced that her positive self-image had merely been a form of vanity that she created as a way of avoiding her "true self." She even suggested that her vanity might be the real reason her marriage broke apart.

As far as I could tell, Sheila's medical crisis, her belief in a painful past that she could not uncover, and her deteriorating self-image actually created more of a dilemma than the breakup of her marriage. Yet she was resurrecting grief over her divorce, instead of admitting that her husband's leaving could have been caused by a constellation of his own issues. By subordinating her health problems to her search for elusive negative past experiences and to grieve over her marriage, she may have been allowing her breast cancer to worsen, along with her self-image.

What Sheila could have done, as many people do, is confront the myth that their lives are entirely under their own control and eventually dismiss it entirely from their psyches.

Questions for Self-Examination

+ Are you always searching for what you did to deserve your illness?

+ Do you believe that until you uncover what you did wrong, you won't be able to heal?

+ Do you find yourself dwelling on negative experiences from the past, believing that doing this actually enhances your healing?

THE FIFTH MYTH: TRUE CHANGE IS IMPOSSIBLE

The final myth is especially debilitating because it has a great deal of clout within the psyche regardless of whether one is physically ill. The reason we believe change is impossible is simple: No one likes change, and no one likes *to* change. We like everything to remain familiar—perversely enough, even in very difficult situations. We believe that "the devil we know is better than the one we don't," and that's how most of us look at the process of change.

Even though change is constant and inevitable, we prefer to turn our attention—and a great deal of our attention—to preventing changes from happening in our lives. Suggesting to people that they initiate change and call upon the winds to pull their ship from its safe harbor into the moving seas is akin to asking them to sit on hot coals for an afternoon. Yet the truth is that healing and change are one and the same thing. They are composed of the same energy, and we cannot seek to heal an illness without first looking into what behavioral patterns and attitudes need to be altered in our life. Once those characteristics are identified, we have to do something about those patterns. This requires taking action, and action brings about change.

Many people convince themselves that quitting an addiction or beginning a routine of bodywork represents sufficient change for healing to occur. Certainly these changes support healing, but quite frankly they contribute very little to the real issues that may be preventing healing. Healing requires internal as well as external change. It requires asking ourselves questions such as "Am I fulfilled by the life I am leading? Have I given enough attention to my own personal needs, or have I just sought to look after the needs of others?" These questions not only direct our attention to ourselves but also compel us to shift directions in our lives and even change our nature. At this point, we usually begin to argue with ourselves, telling ourselves again and again that we simply cannot change our natures. "This is the way I have always been," we say, "because this is who I am."

The myth that true change is impossible is entrenched within us as deeply as our DNA. Everything and everyone seems to support it because we don't want to change ourselves any more than we believe others can change. Even when we are holding out hope that someone will change his or her negative characteristics, we usually doubt that this kind of transformation can actually be accomplished.

To work change into the depths of our nature, we need to come to grips with those characteristics within us that we have tended to avoid. We are often completely unaware of certain parts of our personalities, either because we do not want to recognize them or because we have never given much attention to our shadow side. Regardless of the reason, we must face them once and for all. It is not an easy task. We don't like diving into our dark side, and we don't like bringing our fears and negative qualities out into the open.

At one of my workshops, a 41-year-old woman named Louisa told her story of dealing with ovarian cancer. She had sought out the assistance of a therapist trained in hypnosis. Initially, the hypnotic treatments seemed ineffectual, mainly because Louisa could not relax enough to allow her mind to turn off. One day the therapist suggested that before their next appointment Louisa get a massage. She did, after which she arrived at her therapist's office slightly more relaxed—enough to allow her to go under. During hypnosis Louisa began to speak about her fear of aging. She believed that aging represented the loss of her beauty, her sexual attractiveness, and therefore her power as a woman. She spoke of aging as a disease that had no cure, saying that every part of her preferred death to living as an elderly woman who had to look at the faces of younger and more attractive women.

When the therapist shared these revelations after Louisa came out of trance, her response was complete denial. "How can I fear aging? After all, it's a natural part of life. Everyone ages."

In the next session the therapist showed Louisa fashion magazines filled with photographs of beautiful women. She asked Louisa to comment on how beautiful the models were. With each page Louisa became increasingly uncomfortable, remarking that underneath all that makeup these women were just ordinary people. Yet her tension mounted as her therapist asked her to imagine what life must be like for women of such beauty. She said that she had no idea. And then her therapist asked her if she thought any of these women had a fear of aging.

"Of course they do," Louisa said. "How could they not? Their face is their fortune, and when that goes, so does their career and their personal life. No man wants an old woman."

"You are talking about yourself," her therapist responded, "and you need to realize that. This fear is so deep inside of you that you are destroying your female organs because you so resent the aging process taking place within your female body."

Louisa insisted that there was absolutely no connection between her illness and this "fabricated" fear of aging. From her point of view, her cancer was the result of stress from her job, or maybe just her bad luck. Louisa could not open herself to even considering the possibility of another interpretation of her crisis. For her, a change in perspective was impossible—she would only change her life in ways that did *not* change her image of herself.

At the other end of this spectrum, some people regard internal change as not only possible but as a bit of an adventure, especially when they approach it with a sense of humor. Linda, a woman who had to cope with skin cancer, was absolutely delightful, full of humor and warmth. She decided to look at her healing as an adventure, commenting, "I always wanted to go exploring, but I sure as hell never thought it would be inside of me!"

Linda was open to any and all forms of healing on the market. After investigating many therapeutic possibilities, she met a man who was both a therapist and a meditation teacher. They got together twice a week, and as she said to me, "When we weren't on the outside, we were on the inside." As part of her therapy, he directed Linda to enter a meditative state and then answer his questions. To help herself cooperate completely with him, she created a poem that she would repeat a few times before she relaxed into a meditative state: "In I go, off to mend; out I come, healthy again."

"Since it was something I knew I needed to do," she told me, "I thought that I would be much better off working with it than working against it. I never knew that I was afraid of becoming close to people, but I was. And I found out that I had a real phobia about closed-in spaces, a fear of not being able to get out of locked rooms. I suspect that is why I spent so much time outdoors, and all that sun was probably not good for me. My therapist pointed out that both these fears revolved around closeness.

Now I talk to myself whenever I'm in a closed room, telling myself that I'm not afraid of this anymore. I also tell myself that if any other fears are hanging out in me, to come on up and show themselves. I'm ready for anything now."

We rarely think that changing ourselves could be an adventure, but why should it not? Illness is associated so closely with fears and negative patterns that we can become as frightened of healing ourselves as we are of the disease itself. The knowledge of how much and how deeply we need to change is as intimidating as it is true. Linda's remarkable attitude offers a positive option of a lighthearted approach to healing, as unlikely and as difficult as it may appear.

When Larry was coping with migraines, high blood pressure, and an ulcer, he finally reached the point where he had had enough of living in a "deteriorating body," as he put it. He felt that he had become a "physical slum," and that he was the "landlord of a feudal system that needed to be modernized."

Larry put together a healing program that covered all the bases: physical, mental, emotional, and spiritual. Mainly, though, he focused on his emotional problems, which he felt formed the core of his toxicity. I got a kick out of Larry because he was one of the few men I had ever met who actually went for a makeover, the way some women do. As a part of his healing, so that he could understand the weaknesses and gaps in his emotional nature, he met with many of his women friends and former romantic partners and asked each one how she viewed him and the way he expressed his emotions.

Next, he went to a therapist and handed her the list of qualities that the women had frankly identified. These included a self-centered nature, a lack of compassion for others, an out-of-control temper, and a tendency to exaggerate things in order to get more attention than anyone else. Once Larry had gotten over the shock of seeing how he came across to women, he and his therapist went to work on him.

"At first," he said, "I felt as if we were attempting to climb a mountain that had no peak but just kept going on and on—or should I say, digging a pit that had no bottom. I have to admit that I felt embarrassed by what these women had said about me. If I were ever to do something like this again, I would at least ask them to say something—anything—positive, too, to soften the blow. At any rate, my therapist directed me to think about my childhood to see if I could find the source of my self-centeredness. That's when I realized that I was always looking for attention from my parents—and even though they gave me a great deal of love and attention, it was never enough. I always wanted more, and this need continued throughout my adulthood. At one point, I told my therapist that I was beginning to think of myself as a pretty lousy human being, but she just laughed and told me that was an indication that we were on the right path. I still don't know what she meant by that remark, but I did keep working with her."

Because of Larry's enthusiasm and fearless self-investigation, he noticed that his body was releasing more and more tension. His migraines didn't stop right away, but his blood pressure returned to normal and his ulcer began to heal. To help him cope with his migraines, his therapist introduced him to biofeedback, which is known to be effective with migraines because it helps a person direct attention to sending warmth into the hands, which tends to release the pressure in the brain.

"Simultaneously with all this therapeutic work," Larry concluded, "I wanted to become a different kind of person, if only to keep myself healthy. I suppose that decision was also self-centered, but who cares? It worked. Whenever I was out on a date or with a friend, I no longer talked just about myself. I asked them how they were doing, and I worked to be a better listener. At first I was trying to impress them with my new self, but I soon found that I was actually interested in what everyone had to say. And most of all, I really liked the person I was becoming." Not surprisingly, Larry soon healed his migraines, along with everything else.

Our belief that we are damaged at our core is accompanied by the belief that we are not worthy of any kind of help, human or Divine, or of acting on any of the help offered to us. Cutting loose from this emotional anchor takes real effort. The effort required is not superhuman, however; as Larry showed, it just takes will. I deeply admire the way Larry took charge of his personality. He seemed to have little fear of his own interior, so much so that he asked for the kind of feedback that many of us would have found too difficult to deal with. But no obstacle was large enough to deflect Larry from his goal. And though healing migraines is small change compared with healing cancer, I'm not so sure that it would have made much difference to Larry, in terms of his approach. I believe he would have beaten any illness, or at least given it a good run for its money.

Questions for Self-Examination

+ Do you think about change more than you act to bring it about?

+ Do you always imagine that change will be troublesome and depressing rather than adventuresome or exciting?

+ Do you think of change as something that will make your life feel out of control and chaotic?

I have rarely, if ever, met a person who does not believe at least one of these five myths. Because they are so rampant, breaking free of them and the thought and behavior patterns that accompany them is very hard work. You should be comforted, however, to know that this is not a road you walk alone. The path is more crowded than you can imagine, and most of your companions find it as challenging as you do. As a starting point for healing, try some of the positive methods described in this chapter. Add whatever other methods you feel will assist you in making the important internal changes that support your healing.

Don't fear the despair or exhaustion that you will inevitably feel along the way. No one can remain positive and strong all the time, not even under the best of circumstances. Books can make healing sound as if there's nothing to it—just change your mind, get positive, get active, and eat right. Would that it were that simple! But it is not. Again and again, you need to look inside, confront the myths in which you believe, and clear out your fears and negative patterns. You need to continue to practice this even after you heal. Even though you are not to blame for your illness, you will need to look within to learn to cope with it, find meaning in it, live with and through it, and heal it. Where else have we to look? We can stare at the heavens, but ultimately we are always in our bodies. We wonder about our place in the scheme of things, we wonder about the nature of God, we wonder about the length of our lives. Are these questions really any different from the ones we ask when we do our internal work, when we search for our own negativity, or for those parts of ourselves that we have ignored for far too many years? In truth, we have no choice but to move ever more closely into ourselves—the only way out, as the expression goes, is to go in.

You can take comfort from the fact that illness is not the only way we can make contact with and eliminate the fears underlying the five myths; it is simply one of the most forcible. Life itself is a journey through these myths, and at various times along the way we have to confront the same fears, whether during a career crisis, a marriage falling apart, the death of a loved one, or even a sudden success, which may fill us with the fear that our friends will become envious and abandon us. Every experience in life draws us into ourselves, for whether we succeed or fail, we will ask ourselves if we are getting better or worse and then wonder about which part within us is most affected or changed. Illness demands that you turn inward and become conscious of yourself.

Chapter Three

THE CHAKRAS,
THE ASTROLOGICAL AGES,
AND THE FORMS
OF POWER

The stunning transformations in attitudes and beliefs about healing that have occurred in the last few decades have clearly been difficult for many of us to integrate into our lives. One way to put these changes in perspective and become a little more comfortable navigating them is to look at them in the context of the arc of historical development that has led up to them. Since I view history through the lens of spiritual as well as physical and technological progress, I will also briefly look at the system of human energy as defined by the chakras, which is at the core of my beliefs about healing. From there, I will proceed to examine the relationship between the last three astrological ages and the particular manifestations of human psychospiritual power that have developed in each of them.

THE CHAKRAS

Knowledge of the chakras has existed for thousands of years, although only in the last century has it filtered through to the West in any great detail. According to the Hindu and Buddhist metaphysical systems, the seven chakras are the traditional energy centers of the astral body, a subtle energy plane that coexists with the physical body. The chakras are the areas of interconnection between body and spirit that, when purified or opened up through the advanced practices of yoga, lead the adept to enlightenment—although in certain people, for reasons that are not entirely clear, the chakras may sometimes open spontaneously. They are often pictured as lotus blossoms or spinning wheels (in Sanskrit, *chakra* means "wheel" or "circle"), and each subtle chakra roughly corresponds to a location in the physical body. (A similar system, with different terminologies, is employed by some schools of Taoism in China.)

The first, or Muladhara chakra, lies at the point between the anus and the genitals where the vital energy of body and spirit resides like a coiled serpent. In the Hindu system, the process of uncoiling that serpent is known as Kundalini Yoga. The second chakra lies at the root of the genitals; the third corresponds to the solar plexus; the fourth is located near the heart (either in the middle of the chest or closer to the right side); the fifth is in the throat region; the sixth is located slightly behind the space between the eyebrows (the so-called third eye); the seventh is located just above the crown of the head, although it corresponds to the pineal gland. This last chakra is called the Sahasrara chakra, from the Sanskrit word for "thousand," referring to the "thousand-petaled lotus" of enlightenment. There is also an eighth chakra that exists outside of the physical body, at the upper edge of the auric field, but I will save my discussion of that chakra for Chapter 7.

For those in the West who are unfamiliar with Eastern terminology and metaphysics, it may be simpler to think of the chakras as computer disks that are imprinted with information of all sorts. Much like the hard disk in your computer, the chakras spin and take in data and also can be tapped to disgorge that same information. Each energy data bank resonates to a very specific vibration of energy needed by your physical and spiritual body.

SEVEN POWER CENTERS OR CHAKRAS OF THE KUNDALINI SYSTEM

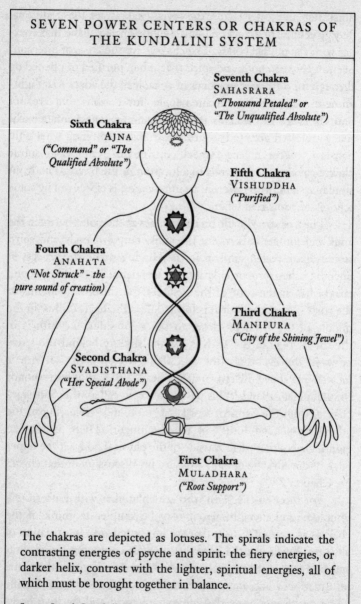

Seventh Chakra
SAHASRARA
("Thousand Petaled" or
"The Unqualified Absolute")

Sixth Chakra
AJNA
("Command" or "The
Qualified Absolute")

Fifth Chakra
VISHUDDHA
("Purified")

Fourth Chakra
ANAHATA
("Not Struck" - the
pure sound of creation)

Third Chakra
MANIPURA
("City of the Shining Jewel")

Second Chakra
SVADISTHANA
("Her Special Abode")

First Chakra
MULADHARA
("Root Support")

The chakras are depicted as lotuses. The spirals indicate the contrasting energies of psyche and spirit: the fiery energies, or darker helix, contrast with the lighter, spiritual energies, all of which must be brought together in balance.

Source: Joseph Campbell, *The Mythic Image* (Princeton, N.J.: Princeton University Press, 1974)

According to the Eastern understanding, the universal life-force flows through the top of the head and down the chakras, nurturing our bodies with seven distinct kinds of energy, each essential to our physical and spiritual development. And it flows upward through the chakras, communicating individual insight and a conscious sense of universal interconnectedness.

Although all the chakras are an inherent part of our spiritual and physical makeup, I believe that human beings have only gained full access to each of them during different phases of our psychospiritual evolution. Similarly, as each of us grows from infancy to adulthood, we activate the chakras' energies and spiritual lessons in sequence from bottom to top. Here is a thumbnail description of some of the belief patterns and behaviors associated with each of the chakras, in ascending order. You may want to refer back to these descriptions as we discuss the relationship of the chakras to the astrological ages and the forms of power in the rest of this chapter.

> *First chakra:* This energy center contains the belief patterns most strongly connected to our biological family and our early social environment. The identifying characteristic of first chakra patterns is that they are group thought-forms, stemming from religious, ethnic, cultural, social, business, political, and family traditions. These patterns teach tribal members either how to take control of groups or how to relinquish control to group authority figures, and thus the spiritual challenges of this chakra relate to how well we manage our physical world.

> *Second chakra:* From group control, we move to control on a one-to-one basis. Second chakra patterns and lessons apply most strongly to sexual relationships, friendships, business and financial partnerships and power, and any other kind of one-on-one interaction that brings out the need to take charge of a situation. Control patterns, of course, include both positive and negative expressions of behavior, and everyone

Energy Anatomy

CHAKRA	ORGANS
1	Physical body support
	Base of spine
	Legs, bones
	Feet
	Rectum
	Immune system
2	Sexual organs
	Large intestine
	Lower vertebrae
	Pelvis
	Appendix
	Bladder
	Hip area
3	Abdomen
	Stomach
	Upper intestines
	Liver, gallbladder
	Kidney, pancreas
	Adrenal glands
	Spleen
	Middle spine

MENTAL, EMOTIONAL ISSUES	PHYSICAL DYSFUNCTIONS	
Physical family and group safety and security	Chronic lower back pain	**1**
Ability to provide for life's necessities	Sciatica	
Ability to stand up for self	Varicose veins	
Feeling at home	Rectal tumors/cancer	
Social and familial law and order	Depression	
	Immune-related disorders	
Blame and guilt	Chronic lower back pain	**2**
Money and sex	Sciatica	
Power and control	Ob/gyn problems	
Creativity	Pelvic/low back pain	
Ethics and honor in relationships	Sexual potency	
	Urinary problems	
Trust	Arthritis	**3**
Fear and intimidation	Gastric or duodenal ulcers	
Self-esteem, self-confidence, and self-respect	Colon/intestinal problems	
	Pancreatitis/diabetes	
Care of oneself and others	Indigestion, chronic or acute	
Responsibility for making decisions	Anorexia or bulimia	
Sensitivity to criticism	Liver dysfunction	
Personal honor	Hepatitis	
	Adrenal dysfunction	

Energy Anatomy (cont'd)

CHAKRA	ORGANS
4	Heart and circulatory system
	Lungs
	Shoulders and arms
	Ribs/breasts
	Diaphragm
	Thymus gland
5	Throat
	Thyroid
	Trachea
	Neck vertebrae
	Mouth
	Teeth and gums
	Esophagus
	Parathyroid
	Hypothalamus
6	Brain
	Nervous system
	Eyes, ears
	Nose
	Pineal gland
	Pituitary gland

MENTAL, EMOTIONAL ISSUES	PHYSICAL DYSFUNCTIONS	
Love and hatred	Congestive heart failure	**4**
Resentment and bitterness	Myocardial infarction (heart	
Grief and anger	attack)	
Self-centeredness	Mitral valve prolapse	
Loneliness and commitment	Cardiomegaly	
Forgiveness and compassion	Asthma/allergy	
Hope and trust	Lung cancer	
	Bronchial pneumonia	
	Upper back, shoulder	
	Breast cancer	
Choice and strength of will	Raspy throat	**5**
Personal expression	Chronic sore throat	
Following one's dream	Mouth ulcers	
Using personal power to create	Gum difficulties	
Addiction	Temporomandibular joint	
Judgment and criticism	problems	
Faith and knowledge	Scoliosis	
Capacity to make decisions	Laryngitis	
	Swollen glands	
	Thyroid problems	
Self-evaluation	Brain tumor/hemorrhage/	**6**
Truth	stroke	
Intellectual abilities	Neurological disturbances	
Feelings of adequacy	Blindness/deafness	
Openness to the ideas of others	Full spinal difficulties	
Ability to learn from experience	Learning disabilities	
Emotional intelligence	Seizures	

Energy Anatomy (cont'd)

CHAKRA	ORGANS
7	Muscular system
	Skeletal system
	Skin

experiences some form of negative one-to-one control patterns in their lives that need to be confronted in terms of the influence these patterns have on their energy and their bodies.

Third chakra: This energy center relates most strongly to the belief patterns we hold about ourselves, including our physical appearance, intelligence, physical abilities, and skills, from athletics to dancing to quilt-making. In short, this chakra is the center of our self-esteem, and, as such, the spiritual challenges related to this center concern the maturation of the ego.

Fourth chakra: The heart-center of the human body is the generator of all emotions: love, kindness, jealousy, anger, hatred. The heart can be considered the most powerful of all the chakras because it has utter authority to create or destroy; as such, heart energy may also be the most challenging to master. If your heart energy is managed by Tribal power, then your emotional connections will be limited accordingly. The spiritual challenges of the fourth chakra are to learn compassion, the value of forgiveness, and the meaning of conscious love, often referred to as "uncondi-

MENTAL, EMOTIONAL ISSUES	PHYSICAL DYSFUNCTIONS	
Ability to trust life	Energetic disorders	**7**
Values, ethics, and courage	Mystical depression	
Humanitarianism	Chronic exhaustion that is not linked to a physical disorder	
Selflessness		
Ability to see the larger pattern	Extreme sensitivities to light, sound, and other environmental factors	
Faith and inspiration		
Spirituality and devotion		

tional love," which makes the heart a universal instrument of goodness without private agendas that can reduce love to acts of manipulation and attempts to control others.

Fifth chakra: This energy center is the center of human willpower, the place from which we speak our truth. Every choice we make carries the power to ignite change. The more conscious you become that there is no such thing as private choice, the more impact your will has. The spiritual challenge of this chakra is to recognize that your strength of will is measured not by how well you exert your will over others, which is our cultural tendency, but by how well you control yourself. Conscious self-control and discipline means living according to the truth that every thought you have is either a potential act of grace or a potential weapon. Right thought leads to right speech leads to right acting. You need to learn to direct your life-force consciously into the kinds of thoughts that will return positive energy to you. This rule becomes even more crucial when you are facing an illness. Alternative healing techniques in particular require that your will be aligned with your heart to produce effective results. Without this strength of will, visualization and other internal disciplines carry only the power of sweet daydreams, not the force required to effect a shift in your physical biology.

Sixth chakra: This energy center runs the power of the mind. As the core of your consciousness, it carries tremendous authority. A spiritual truth is that reality exists behind our eyes, not in front of them, and this chakra challenges us to become familiar with deeper levels of being and consciousness. Each one of us will repeatedly be challenged to reconsider beliefs in which we have invested energy. At times, we will realize that these beliefs are empty of meaning, and we will need to learn other, truer beliefs. The characteristics inherent in the sixth chakra can either be our biggest obstacles or our greatest assets: pride and the ability to make judgments. Used positively, they can lead us to act wisely; in their negative or shadow manifestations, they can lead us into arrogance and cynicism. The spiritual lessons of the sixth chakra relate to insight and intuition, to seeing beyond the visible.

Seventh chakra: The energy of this center is like a magnet that draws us upward into Divine perception. It provides us with hope and faith. It is what I call our "grace bank account" or our "cellular bank account," warehousing the energy generated by our prayers and other acts of spiritual devotion. It is also our spiritual conscience—the part of us that seeks the company of God, with or without our awareness, reminding us that life is about more than the acquisition of goods. If you can learn to be conscious of the subtle Divine current flowing through this chakra, it will generate the transforming spiritual quests and questions of your life: For what purpose was I born? What is truth? What is the deeper meaning of life, and can I find that? Failure to hear and respond to these questions can lead to feelings of anxiety and depression.

The Chakras, the Sacraments, and the Tree of Life

There are many ways to chart our spiritual growth; for me, the combination of the chakras with the symbolic language of the Christian sacraments and the Kabbalistic tradition has proven to be the most useful.

Certain truths are universal in all spiritual traditions: for example, all spiritual systems teach respect for life and personal energy, and that murder and stealing are wrong. But the Hindu, Christian, and Jewish spiritual traditions, in particular, have parallels even greater than these very broad ones. To a remarkable extent, the seven chakras correspond to the symbol systems of the Christian sacraments and the Tree of Life, so that taken together they constitute a journey of spiritual development.

Easiest to see is the correspondence between the seven chakras and the seven Christian sacraments. When the sacraments are lined up in a certain order—Baptism first, then Communion, Confirmation, Marriage, Confession, Ordination, and Extreme Unction (which is now called Anointing the Sick)—their functions remarkably parallel, in meaning and power, those of the seven chakras. (Although my ordering of the sacraments isn't the one that is generally given in the Catholic Church today, it may actually be closer to the order in which the catechumens of the early Church received them.) Both systems illustrate in their own language the dynamic flow of energy that gives life to the human body.

Similarly, in the Kabbalistic tradition, the Tree of Life contains ten qualities of human nature that we need to cultivate for full spiritual maturity. Because six of the ten qualities, or *sefirot*, are counterparts of each other, the Tree of Life actually appears to have seven levels, as in the other two traditions. These three traditions thus seem to offer a slightly different but compatible and harmonizing perspective on the same truth: Spirit evolves through seven distinct stages of power.

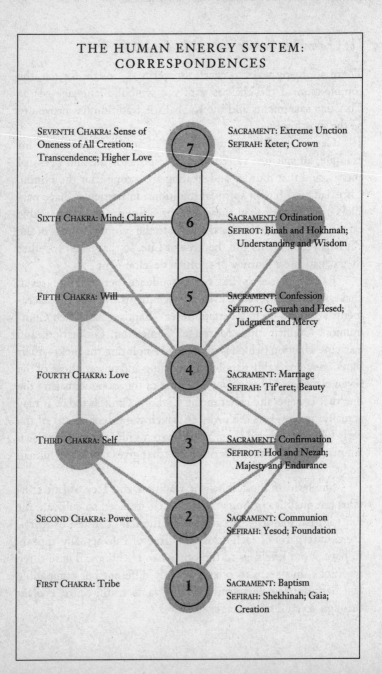

THE HUMAN ENERGY SYSTEM: CORRESPONDENCES

SEVENTH CHAKRA: Sense of Oneness of All Creation; Transcendence; Higher Love

7

SACRAMENT: Extreme Unction
SEFIRAH: Keter; Crown

SIXTH CHAKRA: Mind; Clarity

6

SACRAMENT: Ordination
SEFIROT: Binah and Hokhmah;
Understanding and Wisdom

FIFTH CHAKRA: Will

5

SACRAMENT: Confession
SEFIROT: Gevurah and Hesed;
Judgment and Mercy

FOURTH CHAKRA: Love

4

SACRAMENT: Marriage
SEFIRAH: Tif'eret; Beauty

THIRD CHAKRA: Self

3

SACRAMENT: Confirmation
SEFIROT: Hod and Nezah;
Majesty and Endurance

SECOND CHAKRA: Power

2

SACRAMENT: Communion
SEFIRAH: Yesod; Foundation

FIRST CHAKRA: Tribe

1

SACRAMENT: Baptism
SEFIRAH: Shekhinah; Gaia;
Creation

THE ASTROLOGICAL AGES

The gradual development of our individual spiritual natures through the course of a single lifetime is mirrored in the historical development of human spirituality over many ages. According to an accepted principle of biological evolution, every so often a species makes a quantum leap in its development. I believe that several times in the last four or five thousand years, an equivalent evolutionary leap has happened to humanity on a psychospiritual level. Since my theory about the development of the chakras is based on intuition rather than on provable scientific facts, however, it may be easier for you to think of them as a metaphor for human spiritual evolution. Furthermore, as we prepare to enter the next millennium, I believe we are in the midst of yet another huge jump forward in our spiritual progress.

In my study of Christian scripture over the years, I had occasionally come across astrological symbolism, exemplified most dramatically by the statement in the New Testament that three kings followed a star in the heavens as their sign that a new birth and a great significance had taken place on the earth. As a longtime admirer of the spiritual language and lessons of astrology, I began to explore this interface, and began to see a correlation between the beginning of the traditional astrological ages and the appearance of new spiritual ideas in human consciousness. As each astrological age unfolded itself, new spiritual teachings reshaped our understanding of ourselves, the nature of God and the world, and our place in it. These new patterns of thought become the sources of inspiration behind all cultural changes, redirecting every conscious and unconscious social impulse that is a part of the collective life-force. This astrological-historical context for the emergence of spiritual truths may enhance your understanding of your own spiritual journey and your capacity to heal yourself and your life.

Astrological ages are two-thousand-year cycles. (In strictly astrological parlance, each age begins when the Sun, at the moment of the spring equinox, enters the thirty-degree arc of sky identified by that particular sign of the zodiac.) The three most recent astrological ages are Aries, which ran from about 2000 B.C. to the birth of Christ; Pisces, the current age, which is just about over; and Aquarius, the age we are now entering, which should extend to around the year 4000.

To understand the significance, and the challenges, of the new era we are entering, we first have to understand where we have come from and where we are today.

The Age of Aries: Tribal Power

All twelve signs of the zodiac are associated with one of the major elements: fire, earth, air, or water. Aries is a fire sign, and fire is the element associated with taking action. The characteristics associated with Aries are creativity, leadership, loyalty, motivation, and the capacity to initiate new beginnings. People born under the sign of Aries, by nature, have a "can do" attitude. It was during the age of Aries that Tribal culture was organized, in which the focus of human consciousness was directed toward developing unified tribal communities to achieve physical survival. The goal was to achieve group strength and physical endurance, and to master the external components of life. It was an age not of emotional or psychological introspection, but of learning to manage external challenges.

The new patterns of consciousness that begin with each astrological age serve as that age's ground rules. The age of Taurus, the two-thousand-year period that preceded the Arien age, represented a much cruder form of Tribal culture, without the organizing force of structured laws in many parts of the world and particularly by that part that gave rise to the Western spiritual heritage. During the age of Taurus, sacrifice, including human sacrifice, was viewed as a means of appeasing the wrath of God. But at the dawn of the age of Aries, Abraham received instructions from Yahveh to found the nation of Israel, according to the Book of Genesis in the Bible, and so the Patriarchy of the Jewish people came into being. Prior to the formation of the nation of Israel, the itinerant Hebrews had lived similarly to the Canaanites, practicing animal and human sacrifice.

Considering how commonly human sacrifice occurred then, it would not have been unexpected for Yahveh to instruct Abraham to sacrifice his only son, Isaac. As Abraham and Isaac prepared the sacrificial altar, Isaac was perplexed because he could not see what would be offered to God by his death. Abraham told his son, "God will provide himself the lamb for the burnt offering." After the altar was in place, Abraham bound his son, laid Isaac upon the altar, and prepared to slay him with his knife. An angel appeared to Abraham and stopped him, saying, "Do not lay a hand on the lad or do anything to him; for now I know that you fear God, because you did not withhold your son, your only son, from me." Abraham then looked up and saw a ram caught in a bush, and he offered it to God in lieu of his son (Genesis 22).

This famous episode is traditionally taught in Sunday school as a test of Abraham's obedience to God's will, but its Symbolic meaning is far more significant. In metaphorical terms, the story tells us that humanity had evolved to a position of greater authority with God, such that human sacrifice was no longer required to please God or gain atonement. On yet another level, the shift away from "sacrificial consciousness" suggests that human awareness had expanded sufficiently that humanity itself saw a new, greater value in human life. Our ancestors realized that God had never required human sacrifice; the practice was a reflection of the lesser value that humankind had placed on life as subjects of an external god that they felt they needed to placate.

Following this sacrifice, God told Abraham that his descendants would give birth to the nation of Israel. Sacrifice shifted from an act of appeasement to a sealing of a covenant with God and an expression of gratitude to the heavens. Yet the idea of sacrifice as a means through which guilt is pardoned and holiness restored remains powerful within human consciousness even today. We are still heavily influenced by the belief that the mind of God can be swayed by sacrifice.

Abraham is believed to have lived around 2000 B.C., at the dawn of the age of Aries and of a new order of power for the Hebrew people. His grandson Jacob had twelve sons, from whom came the Twelve Tribes of Israel (a correspondence to the twelve signs of the zodiac). Midway through the Arien age, probably around 1200 B.C., Moses led the Jews from Egypt back to the Promised Land in a journey symbolic of uniting the Hebrew people in their faith in the one God. The Ten Commandments and other tribal laws emerged and formed the basis for what it meant to be a Jew: "Tribal consciousness" was molded into a sense of genuine identity and order. The Hebrew scriptures were also written under Aries, with frequent reference to the covenants with God and the sacrificial lambs used to seal them.

Under Aries, Tribal consciousness became more sophisticated not only for the Jews, but also for the Greeks, Romans, Egyptians, and other cultures of that time. Tribal identity and a sense of nationality—belonging to a single nation rather than just a clan or a tribe—became prominent. The theme of the age of Aries and Tribal culture was dominance and authority over the external environment. The natural sciences, law, and even the Roman system of roads all sprang out of Tribal consciousness.

The earliest Tribal religions worshiped gods who were more or less identified with Nature, and so most Tribal superstitions are designed to try to manage the temperament of the gods by not getting heaven angry. Furthermore, the fearful belief patterns that are inherent in Tribal consciousness remain among the most influential in present-day thinking. One reason may be that they are just so ancient that they are almost genetically programmed into human consciousness.

Tribal laws during this age sought to control people's behavior to facilitate physical survival. The laws given to Moses in the Book of Exodus defined appropriate Tribal responsibilities, from diet to sexual behavior to responsibility for one's family. These responsibilities correspond to the patterns of consciousness of the first, second, and third chakras, which are those most closely aligned to family, money, power, sex, and self-esteem. Even today, Tribal cultures of the Middle East and the Mediterranean rim preserve an emphasis on codes of honor and shame.

The personality attributed to Yahveh at this time was imbued with human characteristics of the highest ideals, which Hebrew law aimed to promote and emulate. The personality of God was an extension of human nature. If we are loving, then God must be all-loving. If we are people of honor and justice, then God must be the ultimate just Being. In the Book of Exodus Yahveh describes Himself as a God of justice, law, and order, a jealous and vengeful God. He demands loyalty and admits to operating according to a material system of reward and punishment. Hebrew law sought to manage jealousy, vengefulness, and the need for justice, all of which are affinities of the first three chakras. Many people still believe—not rationally, but in their Tribal "gut"—that God rewards good behavior financially and punishes negative behavior the same way.

As humanity has become more conscious of our spiritual capacities, we have elevated our spiritual conception of God. Our expansion of our consciousness has led us to widen our vision of our own potential divinity, power, and humanity. Yet we still rarely overcome the traits of Tribal consciousness—those parts of ourselves that respond instinctively rather than reasonably or Symbolically. These tendencies have serious effects on our health. Jealousy, greed, the desire for vengeance, and other lower-chakra issues remain among the leading emotional factors contributing to the loss of health and our inability to heal. Regardless of how much we *know* we should not be jealous of others, we still cannot halt the gut sensations generated by jealousy. Reason—a skill aligned to our sixth chakra—is often no match for our Tribal consciousness functions.

Moreover, we remain deeply enmeshed in the belief that to speak with God and be heard by God, we must engage in sacrificial dialogue. A woman at one of my workshops revealed that upon learning that her daughter had cancer, she gave up meat and certain other food products, hoping that these actions would "inspire" God to heal her daughter. This woman believed that intercessory prayer alone would not be a strong enough action; she had to take physical action to give prayer enough backbone. Tribal consciousness requires physical action, and this woman's entire identity rested on her role as a matriarch. She prayed publicly, representing the entire family, "becoming" their unified "voice" as a Tribal leader, even admitting that she had to be the one to offer sacrifice, since none of the other family members was strong enough to maintain the discipline.

A biological tribe's duties include acceptance of all new members and educating them in the skills of survival, according to the tribe's standards and laws. Tribal control of life in the external world for physical and financial survival is necessary. Lessons about responsibility are an essential part of preparing to live a successful adult life. Yet we need to learn to distinguish the good parts from the bad in our Tribal heritage. The process of spiritual development challenges us to retain the Tribal influences that are positive and to discard those that are not.

All types of tribes, including business and social organizations, are governed by a code of education for survival, however diluted it may be. Unlike biological tribes, social groups do not have a responsibility to accept new members unconditionally, but they do have an unwritten ethical commitment to introduce new members to the codes and skills essential for that particular group's survival—and for survival within the group. These skills often include codes of dress and behavior and a respect for hierarchy. If a new member does not adopt the proper behavior, he or she remains an outsider and eventually leaves in search of another tribe in which to become assimilated and share power.

There are positive aspects to Tribal power apart from basic survival. Tribal power cultivates loyalty, ethics, and a code of honor, and we see the danger to our society when those are lacking; so many children today are completely dysfunctional because their family has no ethical strength and no honor. They don't know where to turn, so they join gangs in some cases, because at least the gang offers ritual and an honor code of sorts. The danger in Tribal loyalty, of course, is that it has to be attached to the Tribe at all times; loyalty to oneself is a very low priority on the Tribal list.

No matter how much we like to think we have evolved beyond Tribal consciousness, strong elements of it are still at work within all of us. I have taken the same vow most of you probably have at some time: "I will never be like my ———." In my case it was my grandmother. She was the sort of person who, when you went to her home for dinner, wouldn't let you serve yourself; she served you, and she always put a huge mound of food on your plate. After you did the right thing and ate it all, she would put another mountain of food there. When the family started to moan collectively, loosen their belts, and complain that they couldn't eat any more, Grandma would invariably say, "After all I cooked for you today?"

So I vowed I would never, ever be like her. But some years back when I was living in New Hampshire, one night I had some friends over for dinner. As the meal wound down, I actually heard myself say, "Is that all you're going to eat? After all I cooked for you today?"

The words were barely out of my mouth when I excused myself, went in the kitchen, and called my mother. "I'm possessed," I said, and told her what had happened and what I had said without thinking.

My mother listened calmly and then asked, "Did you actually put more food on their plates?"

"No," I said, "I didn't do that."

"Okay, then," Mom said. "You're not possessed. She's just in your kitchen."

We should not underestimate the health consequences of maintaining Tribal consciousness. Symbolically, the immune system does for the physical body precisely what Tribal power does for the group: it protects it from potentially harmful external influences. Since Tribalism resonates with our first, second, and third chakras, the stress generated in our systems through superstitious fear patterns also attacks the physical systems that are connected to these three chakras: our immune system, sexual organs, colon, pancreas, gallbladder, liver, legs, and thighs. Yet a healthy identification and relationship with your family of origin can be a source of emotional and psychological strength, and a firm base for the next level of personal power and individuation.

The Age of Pisces: Individual Power

Pisces is a water sign, and water is the astrological element associated with emotion and introspection. The particular characteristics associated with the astrological age of Pisces, which began about two thousand years ago, are emotional consciousness, intuitive thought, and dualism. The symbol of Pisces—two fish swimming in opposite directions—represents more sophisticated choices and more complicated thought processes. Under Tribal consciousness, individuals allowed—and still allow—the Tribe to make important choices for them, from marriage partners to occupations. The emergence of individual choice during Pisces signaled an entirely new paradigm and, with it, a new perceptual system: Individual power.

To manage this new Individual power under Pisces, the boundaries determining an individual's emotional and mental life had to be defined with unprecedented formality. The global culture came to embody these same boundaries and definitions of individual and collective roles. Today, many of us see these definitions as stereotypes, but they remain as potent at the individual level as they do at the global. Some of these boundaries are summarized in the two columns below:

CHAKRAS, ASTROLOGICAL AGES, AND FORMS OF POWER   75

MALE ENERGY	FEMALE ENERGY
Western culture	Eastern culture
State power	Church power
Science	Religion
Parent	Child
Reason	Intuition
Mind	Heart
Body	Soul
Aggressiveness	Passivity
External control	Internal control
Independence	Dependence

During the Piscean age, human evolution began the long journey out of the Tribal mind and toward development of the self—allowing individuals to form a separate identity while still to some extent remaining under Tribal influences. Piscean culture also encouraged the growth of all that the self could discover, notably science and medicine. This emphasis on the development of human intelligence became the leading weapon against the superstitious core of Tribal perception and ultimately led to the Enlightenment and to today's secular culture. Because of Piscean energy, human reasoning abilities and emotional energy were given a much greater license to develop.

Western romance was also born under Pisces, from courtly love to the notion that people should be free to marry the partner they love rather than submit to marriages arranged by Tribal elders. (Even today, however, within many Tribal cultures, it is a given that the tribe will choose one's life partner.) The story of Romeo and Juliet became the archetypal drama of individuals' desires to follow their own emotional needs in contradiction to Tribal and familial custom. Especially in these last centuries, the age of Pisces has clearly given authority over from the tribe to the mind and the heart of humanity.

The history of Western culture under Pisces is symbolic of the step-by-step progress of the power of Individual choice, which took perhaps its most spectacular leap during the Renaissance, when the talents of individual artists extended far beyond the particular "Tribal schools," or workshops of the masters, where they learned their craft. Michelangelo, Raphael, and Leonardo da Vinci led the way, signaling a shift in power in which the individual artist signed his work with his own name rather than with the name of the school for which he painted or leave it unsigned as an act of submersion in the Tribal talent pool. The self as artist, author, or musician—or all three—was born.

Eastern culture was initiated into this new energy pattern through the birth of Gautama the Buddha. The Buddha was born around 500 B.C., roughly three-quarters of the way through the age of Aries, but the growth of Buddhism took place in three distinct periods, of which the first shared certain characteristics of Arien energy. The first era, or "turning of the wheel" in Buddhist parlance, is known as Theravada or Hinayana Buddhism and dominated the first five hundred years of Buddhism. Theravada was characterized by practices of renunciation of all earthly possessions and a life of strict separation from any personal human bonding. Reflecting the fire elements of Aries and the law-and-order quality of that age, the strict code of behavioral disciplines that made up Theravada doctrine did not recognize emotional needs as anything more than obstacles to being in the present moment.

At the beginning of the age of Pisces, the Buddhist tradition experienced an enormous revolution—we could call it a Piscean revolution—giving birth to the second turning of the wheel, known as the Mahayana tradition. Buddhism now began to focus on compassion by developing the concept of the bodhisattva, the enlightened individual who vows not to rest until all other beings have also become enlightened. Although Theravada insisted that only ordained male monks could experience enlightenment and nirvana, Mahayana allowed that laymen and women could too. The third turning of the wheel, known as Vajrayana, extended the compassionate orientation of Mahayana, adding more advanced and complex spiritual techniques in order to accelerate the enlightenment of all beings. Of all the Buddhist traditions, Mahayana is the one most widely followed in the world today.

The Buddha's teachings undermined the Tribal survival mentality of the Arien age by stressing that trying to protect the ego through violence or by amassing material goods results in human suffering. Prior to the Piscean age, humanity had not cared emotionally for others who were not blood members of the tribe, and physical survival was still the main objective. The Buddha brought humanity more refined lessons in personal development, or Individual power, representing the next step in human spiritual evolution, although his teachings had to wait until the second turning of the wheel, at the start of the Piscean age, to achieve their most other-directed form. From the point of view of human consciousness, the development of compassion toward people who were not blood Tribal members represented an expansion of the overall value of life itself.

The coming of the Christian era has been referred to as the opening of the heart of humanity. Toward that end, Jesus of Nazareth provided a new emotional vocabulary, speaking about love, brotherhood, kindness, and forgiveness—lessons of the heart that each individual must experience. The relationship Jesus had to his "Father" in heaven introduced into Israelite culture a level of intimacy with God that had never before existed. Within Tribal consciousness, one would not dare to address God as "Father"—much less "Daddy," as the Aramaic term *Abba* that Jesus used could be more accurately rendered. In assuming that God took a loving interest in every area of one's personal life, Jesus initiated the parent-child relationship between humanity and heaven and gave individuals the means to establish a closer union with the Divine. In time, Mary, the Mother of God, became the Christian version of the "Divine Mother Goddess."

The crucifixion and death of Jesus introduced two major themes of the Piscean age: compassion for all, including those outside the Tribe, and forgiveness. One of the greatest struggles of the healing process is to forgive both yourself and others and to stop expending valuable energy on past hurts. More than any other teacher, Jesus epitomized this spiritual advance through his words on the cross in behalf of the very people who were killing him: "Father, forgive them, for they know not what they do."

Yet for all the centuries that Christianity has been a part of human consciousness, we have still to master forgiveness, or even reach a mild comfort level with it. Part of the reason for our inability may be that although forgiveness makes sense to us intellectually, it makes no sense to our emotional nature and is in conflict with our residual Tribal consciousness. On one level it seems to offend our sense of justice, as if we were saying to someone who has hurt us, "That's all right. What you did to me doesn't matter." We feel that a crime against us must be punished—or that *we* must be punished for our own misdeeds, bad thoughts, or negative attitudes. When we get stuck with these feelings of offense, not only have we failed to understand the meaning of forgiveness and its significance in our spiritual evolution, but we have also missed its importance to our healing.

The other major theme of the age of Pisces is choice, which may well be the only true power that we have. The choices we make throughout our lifetime are our marks of distinction in both the physical and energetic dimensions. Under Tribal consciousness, our power to choose is controlled by the group's perceptions. We see what the group sees, believe as the group believes, love what the group loves, and hate what the group hates. While this may give us a sense of security, it inhibits the development of our ability to think for ourselves.

Jesus embodied the power of choice during his lifetime as recorded in the New Testament, challenging the Tribal elders of his faith and offering the people an alternative approach to God, to each other, and to the crises that fill every life. On the day before his death, Jesus went to the garden of Gethsemane to pray with his disciples. As the disciples fell into a deep sleep, Jesus prayed to God, "Abba, Father, all things are possible to you; remove this cup from me. Yet not what I will but what you will" (Mark 14:36).

In that profound prayer, Jesus consciously chose to accept his fate. He relinquished his will not to the Tribe but to the will of God in an act that symbolizes complete trust in Divine reason. In agreeing to accept the inevitability of his death, the decision to crucify him that would be made the next day had, in effect, already been made between Jesus and God. The Tribal mind, as such, was never a part of this decision, even though it may have seemed throughout the crucifixion that the people of the Roman and Palestinian tribes were responsible for Jesus' death.

When Judas sold information about Jesus' whereabouts for thirty pieces of silver—the most famous act of betrayal in Western culture—he epitomized Tribal power: the use of money and physical force. During the trial that followed, Herod and Pontius Pilate could not make Jesus behave in any familiar Tribal manner. He would not defend himself, scream that he was innocent, or attempt to bargain. Most significantly of all, he was not frightened or disoriented—they were. Jesus informed the Tribal elders confronting him that they had no power whatsoever over the events that were occurring. In every detail of his trial, Jesus responded in a way that baffled the Tribe—illustrating for us that we have options in the face of even the most unjust circumstances.

In effect, all the events leading to Jesus' death were a celebration of the power of choice that his entire life had represented, especially when he chose to forgive his executioners and did not cry out for vengeance. His greatest act of choice occurred shortly afterward, when he chose his own moment of death, saying, "Father, unto you I commend my spirit. It is finished."

Jesus' life, and the Buddha's, represent that we must all inevitably evolve beyond the Tribal level of consciousness. From the perspective of Piscean culture, Judas' act represents not a betrayal but the closure of a relationship with an older level of consciousness, one that has become alien to Jesus. Part of the message Jesus shows us is how to respond to the signal that we must seek a higher level of consciousness—by surrendering our will to God's will.

In our own lives, when the time comes for us to move beyond an old way of thinking and to give up perceptions that no longer serve our growth, we frequently experience the signal to "take up our bed and walk" as an act of betrayal—a Judas kiss. We may work for a company for many years, for instance, believing that it will provide for us in our retirement, only to become part of corporate downsizing during our middle years. We may marry and count on that partner to be with us through our lifetime, only to discover, twenty years into the marriage, that he or she has fallen in love with someone else.

From an ordinary Tribal point of view, these are acts of betrayal. As long as we think of them as betrayals, we take years to recover from them and we lose incalculable amounts of energy over them. Yet if we can learn to view them Symbolically (as in the chapters that follow), we will see that they are the signal to release the belief patterns of the Tribal mind and evolve to the next level of consciousness.

At the point when we are emerging from Tribal consciousness, we are often, if not always, given the choice to take the "wisdom path." All the signals tell us that the time has come to let go and move on with our lives. Those who heed the signals will be presented with their own challenges, but, more often than not, because we fear change, most of us remain in the old and familiar places, clinging to situations and relationships that have essentially ended. You may, for example, experience a growing desire to leave your job, but even as this desire intensifies, you ignore it because you are unsure of where to go next. You tell yourself that you would make the change if only you knew what lay ahead, if only you had something better lined up. As the tension within you mounts, you fight your desire with more and more self-created rationalizations: "It's not the right time," you tell yourself, or "My job situation is bound to improve if I only give it another chance."

But as the months pass, nothing changes except your mounting anger—not only about your job, but at yourself for not having the courage to do anything about it.

Then the next phase of life has no alternative but to manifest in the "woe path." It's not unlike the consequences of letting a decayed tooth go untreated because you can't face the minor pain and expense of having a cavity filled: You end up having to undergo a much more painful and costly procedure to replace the whole tooth. In the case of leaving your job, the consequences are likely to manifest as illness (usually a chronic condition, such as constant headaches or an ulcer) or what you perceive as a betrayal, like getting fired from the job.

The fear of quitting a job or facing up to a deteriorating marriage is actually fear of taking charge of your own life. Rather than accepting that the day has come to confront your fear, walk into your job, and resign, most of us avoid the fear entirely until some experience forces us to look more closely at ourselves. You may, for instance, resist leaving a marriage that has become counterproductive and spiritually damaging, only to find that you or your spouse will do something—like have an affair—that precipitates a divorce, regardless of your attempts to halt the process. You may risk developing a debilitating or fatal disease should the stress become worse. Or you may be even less fortunate still and simply muddle through what Thoreau called a life of "quiet desperation," leaving the difficult work undone and your spiritual and life potential unrealized.

When you experience an apparent act of betrayal, look closely to see if it may not actually be a "Divine invitation" to let go of the old and discover the new. We will all have Judas experiences. But seen through the lens of higher consciousness, they turn out to be powerful turning points in our lives that can introduce us to an entirely new form of power—the power of the Individual self. From that point of view, the words of Jesus—"Forgive them, for they know not what they do"—are especially meaningful. Ponder the possibility that you may have already agreed, in your own garden of Gethsemane, to move forward, but you needed a push to get going. The people who may seem, at the Tribal level, to be participating in an act of betrayal are, in truth, acting out an agreement you have already made with God. How, then, can you be angry at one of the Lord's messengers? There is nothing for which you need to forgive them, for they have done nothing at all to harm you.

Both Jesus and the Buddha were instrumental in giving form to the Piscean face of God, allowing humanity to see more than the simplistic Lord they had come to know under Aries. Buddhism made compassion an extension of the Divine within us and offered a path through which we could become a part of the tranquil nature of the Universe. Jesus introduced a father-figure whose "personality" is the essence of the fourth chakra, the heart center of the body: loving, forgiving, caring.

Whether you make this journey through Buddhism, Christianity, another religion, or none at all is irrelevant. Each of us will eventually be led to a path of internal development that awakens us to our misconceptions and provides us with the opportunity to utilize the Individual power of choice. Be aware that this awakening will probably clash with the power of the Tribal mind, both within and around you, since the tribe does not encourage independence and Individual consciousness.

If the fish swimming in opposite directions that symbolize Pisces stand for options and choice, they also imply polarity and confrontation. As Pisces gained momentum in the latter half of the second millennium, a tidal wave of revolutions swamped the planet. Tribal authority was challenged by those speaking on behalf of the rights of individuals. Entire nations were born, the United States among them, with visions of becoming safe harbors for individuals seeking freedom of political and religious expression. As Pisces was entering its final two centuries, the Industrial Revolution dawned, bringing with it the belief that any individual "self" could become wealthy, challenging the long-held Tribal belief that one had to be "born to power and wealth."

The influence of Pisces has directed humanity to develop the power associated with the fourth, fifth, sixth, and seventh chakras. Whereas the power of Aries is Tribal and externally focused, in alignment with the energy of our first three chakras, Pisces energy is directed toward our internal selves. Chakras four through seven are calibrated to Piscean energy: the heart, will and choice, the mind, and spiritual life. Prior to the Piscean age, the energies associated with the four highest chakras were dominated by the power of the lower three. Now, as the Piscean age comes to a close, the higher chakras function as a perceptual system independent of the Tribal mind. Ultimately, our Tribal and Individual perceptual abilities are meant to work in harmony with each other. Still, great pain and conflict can be generated when the needs of the heart are at odds with the needs of a group with whom we share a bond.

Many people have shared with me their anguish about leaving the religion in which they grew up to follow a more fulfilling spiritual path. The response from their families is almost always criticism and fear, frequently with the warning that the person is falling under the influence of a cult. One woman told me that when she fell in love with a man of another race and moved in with him, her family cut off contact with her completely. They were so ashamed of her choice of partner that they did not want their friends to know what she had done, and it was easier for them to "shun" her than to explain her actions to the Tribe.

Had she listened to the Tribal elders, of course, the results for her Individual self could have been disastrous, ranging from depression to any number of physical maladies. Forms of emotional and mental anguish that correspond to the stress patterns of the four highest chakras include depression and schizophrenia; the inability to forgive oneself and others; guilt over "betraying" the Tribe; and a variety of spiritual crises based on splitting from Tribal traditions, including the Tribal religion.

The actual physical location of an illness does not necessarily indicate the chakra through which the body is losing power;

breast cancer does not always mean a disturbance of the fourth chakra, for example. For almost all illnesses, the main energy loss begins "below the waist," in the Tribal arena; that initial energy loss may then trigger personal and emotional illnesses that are aligned to the fourth chakra.

Perhaps the best indicator of the irrevocable shift from Tribal to Individual power can be seen in what happened in the United States during the Vietnam War. When a nation declares war upon another, the Tribal assumption is that the entire nation will automatically follow that declaration and, with a few quirky minor defections, throw its full weight behind the war effort. Tribal elders rely on this level of loyalty, and when it works, it can be impressive, as in the Allied efforts of World War II. But by the time the conflict in Vietnam had become a focal point of national attention, Piscean energy had reached its zenith. Just as a light-bulb glows brightest before it burns out, the time had come for the final expression of Individual power before being superseded by Symbolic power.

During the 1960s, the power of the Individual was activated as never before, with hundreds of thousands of people challenging the Tribe's war and, more significantly, refusing to recognize the North Vietnamese as enemies. Tribal power was significantly diminished with that action, and since that time, this nation has never again stood on secure Tribal ground in regard to war. By the time of the Persian Gulf War, the U.S. government had to assure the public that involvement in the war would result in virtually no loss of American lives and would have little economic cost—in other words, no "sacrifice" would be necessary to win. Today our Tribal elders are far more focused on maintaining peace than on sending our young men to fight a war. Far from being of political value to our leaders, war has become a potential liability. Yet other nations around the world are still divided internally in Tribal warfare and brutal suppressions of individual civil rights and religious freedom, as Piscean energy ignites its democratizing effects.

The Age of Aquarius: Symbolic Power

Just as the Tribal or Arien mind has not completely disappeared from the Piscean age, the Piscean mind will still manifest itself in the Aquarian age. But in the late 1950s and early 1960s, two events occurred that represented a global mind-shift and gave millions of people a Divine permission to walk down previously restricted spiritual corridors. In 1959 the invasion of Tibet by the Chinese Communists forced the Dalai Lama to flee his homeland and take up residence in India, where he is still based today (although he has become an active figure on the world stage as well). Just three years later, Pope John XXIII hosted a gathering of cardinals at the Second Vatican Council, where Church leaders worked to bring the Catholic Church into the modern age. Viewing these events literally, one would not immediately draw any connection between them. Yet taken together, and seen from a Symbolic point of view, these two events represent an infusion of mystical spirituality into the mainstream of modern life and signaled the beginning of the merger of Eastern and Western spiritual traditions.

As thousands of Buddhist monks in Tibet were compelled to turn to the outside world for support, many of them offered in exchange the exceedingly rich trove of scriptures and teachings that had been stored in their monasteries. Likewise, one of the unintended consequences of Vatican II was that a large number of religious Roman Catholics, perhaps disillusioned by the Council's liberalization of rules, gave up their clerical orders and reentered lay life. Many of these priests, monks, and nuns had pursued advanced degrees in theology and were privy to the classic writings and teachings of the great Christian mystics, from the Desert Fathers to Hildegard of Bingen, Meister Eckhart, Teresa of Ávila, and John of the Cross. As they found their way back into the mainstream of Western society, they carried these teachings with them and spread them to the public in a way they might never have done had they remained in their relatively cloistered religious lives.

As a result of these seemingly unrelated events, the mystical teachings of both the Eastern and Western spiritual traditions became available to ordinary people. In the mid-1960s this process was further aided in the United States by the lifting of immigration barriers that had been in place since 1917. A wave of Indian masters were able to reach our shores just as the spirit of liberation sweeping the country made American minds receptive to the power of their teachings. At the same time, the Christian churches were experiencing a revolution from within, as women demanded the right to be ordained as priests and ministers, and the laity insisted on more inclusion in both the rituals of the Church and its decision-making processes. This opening of the clerical authority structure had begun centuries earlier with the Protestant Reformation; not long after that, the Reform movement within Judaism had had a similar effect on large numbers of Jews. But in the West, at least, mysticism had remained largely submerged in the popular consciousness. That now changed radically.

Religion may still be essentially Tribal, but in the Piscean transition to Aquarius, it is beginning to operate at a much more conscious level and with unprecedented Individual freedom. Modern spirituality, with its more intimate connection with God, has inspired an inner passion that goes beyond the boundaries of parochial religion. As institutional religion loses ground, spirituality is gaining momentum, a spirituality that is more universalist in orientation than the creeds that preceded it. The New Age has proven itself open to a staggering range of spiritual traditions and practices, and even within mainstream religions the trend toward ecumenism, accepting other paths and traditions as valid and worthy of respect, has accelerated.

Through this shift in focus, the word *consciousness* has come to denote the pursuit of the deepest mystical insights in combination with rationality and freedom. Armed with a vocabulary that was previously restricted to monastics and mystics, Western culture has broken through the boundaries of religion and begun plunging, largely unescorted, into the realm of the sacred. Not only do we want to *know about* the Kundalini experience, reincarnation, meditation, and spiritual ecstasy, we want to *live* them. We want the power of these spiritual teachings to activate our biological tissue; we want to feel the presence of God in our bodies as well as in our minds. We want physical contact with the Divine, matching the level of contact previously enjoyed by saints and mystics of the great traditions.

At around the time these changes were taking place in spirituality and religion, we experienced what I call a global mind implant, a kind of hundredth-monkey syndrome. A new perception became accepted in human consciousness, one that is characteristic of Aquarian energy: the idea that we create our own reality. This single notion inspired an entirely new view of the potential of human power in every part of human life. As we saw in Chapter 1, the corollary of this idea is the belief that we create our own health and can effect our own healing. This perception is characteristic of Aquarian energy because Aquarius is an air sign, and air is the astrological element associated with the mind—new ideas and fresh thought.

Where the Piscean energy, symbolized by two fish swimming in opposing directions, represents the separation of forces, Aquarian energy underlies holism—the need to unite groups of people as well as groups of thought. Aquarian consciousness is holistic by design, meaning that it draws people to view life through the lens of unity rather than the lens of difference and division. Holism, a word invented by South African statesman Jan Christiaan Smuts in 1926, reflects an ancient principle that "all is one," teaching us that we cannot, for instance, heal part of an organism without treating the whole of it. Just so, the holistic health movement seeks to heal illness by addressing not symptoms but the whole organism through diet, exercise, and a wide range of complementary treatments. As we move closer to the Aquarian age, these principles have begun to enter the mainstream of medicine.

Aquarian energy drives us to change every part of our lives, especially where we have become too dependent on the familiar, and to investigate every unknown place we can find, particularly those within ourselves. Aquarian power fuels our exploration of our "higher" selves, or the part of us that is beyond the boundaries of our physical bodies and the daily thrum of life. It embodies an energy that can lift human perception into Symbolic sight. This energy fills us with the sensation that we are exquisitely creative beings with internal resources powerful enough to heal illnesses that have always been considered intractable and to challenge the speed at which we age.

As the Aquarian energy was beginning to make itself felt in the 1960s, it inspired massive social revolution. Not yet familiar with how to use this power internally, we used it externally—in the form of the sexual revolution, the feminist movement, the civil rights and antiwar movements, the counterculture, drug culture, developing a voice that eventually became the psychospiritual revolution. People became inflamed with the need to break away from anything conventional, anything that kept old boundaries firmly in place around the mind and heart. It was the beginning of a transition from *Homo sapiens* to *Homo noeticus*—that is, from beings whose perceptions are controlled by the five senses to beings whose perceptions are based on spiritual insight and vision.

Just as the astrological ages of Aries and Pisces each introduced a new phase of consciousness into the human experience (Tribal and Individual, respectively), the Aquarian age is introducing a belief system that is essentially holistic. It relies on a unity of physical, emotional, psychological, and Symbolic interpretations. Beyond its capacities to inspire us to solve problems differently, holistic consciousness unlocks our ability to see events in Symbolic terms rather than "taking them personally." Aquarian energy is more logical and system-driven than emotional Piscean power. This does not mean that it is unemotional; rather, it takes a practical approach to problem solving. Because of its solution-driven nature, Aquarian energy is drawn to humanitarian causes and the crises of the underdog. The many causes that have surfaced during the past thirty years in behalf of social groups that lacked equal rights are manifestations of Aquarian energy penetrating into the mainstream of society.

Aquarius is the ruler of (an astrological term meaning "in charge of") electricity—and electricity is energy. The symbol of Aquarius is the water-bearer, water being the natural conductor of electrical energy. Symbolically, Aquarian impulses are driving us to understand the very role that energy plays in our lives: how it cooperates with our physical anatomy, how the lack of it can cause illness, and how it can heal us. We are beginning to think of ourselves as energy systems, and we are seeking to understand how our energy systems relate to all other forms of life.

Because of our increasing reliance on the transmission of information, the coming millennium has already been labeled the "information age." Yet information in the sense of data transmission is just a more conventional word for energy. The Internet, E-mail, fax machines, and cable and satellite television are all making real the genuine unification of our global community—in Marshall McLuhan's increasingly apt phrase, the "global village." It makes perfect sense that one of the Chinese government's top priorities in attempting to control its population is to restrict access to the World Wide Web. You don't have to be a New Age believer to see that power is rapidly shifting from a physical force to one of thought and energy, the essence of a computerized society.

As I was doing intuitive readings in the late 1980s, I recognized that I was perceiving information that was far more Symbolic in nature than the more grounded information I had become accustomed to evaluating. Eventually I realized that I had made contact with an eighth chakra, one that was transcendent of the body proper, so to speak. This eighth chakra contains a profile of the archetypal influences that are very much a part of a person's spiritual development and everyday life experiences. (See Chapter 7.)

The more I worked with this archetypal information, the more I realized that Symbolic perceptual abilities are the essence of

Aquarian energy. Our unconscious dimension actually seemed to be pressing to come out into the open. The archetypal agreements we make prior to incarnating—which I refer to as our Sacred Contracts—seemed to have positioned us to heal far more rapidly than any other tool I had so far encountered. This helped explain why, during the past thirty years, numerous psychologists, many inspired by the work of Carl Jung, have done substantial research into archetypes. By making contact with the archetypal realm, we acquired the language by which we could bring into conscious awareness the unconscious realm that is intimately woven into our everyday life patterns. The "child," "wounded healer," "warrior," "wild woman," and "hero," for example, are but a handful of the many archetypes that have been introduced into our therapeutic arena as working "voices" to assist people in understanding the Symbolic choreography behind their very real physical problems.

Symbolic perceptions allow us to see that the real meaning of a crisis lies in showing us what we need to learn about ourselves. To blame the other players in our drama for helping to teach us what we need to learn is the height of foolishness. If, for example, I need to learn what it feels like to have something stolen from me, then anyone capable of stealing will do as my teacher. Spending my life resenting a particular "teacher"—waiting for the moment when I can punish the thief or make him or her feel guilty for all my years of mourning my loss—ultimately interferes with my learning process. No one has understood this principle better than the Dalai Lama, who has repeatedly said that he is grateful to the Chinese for forcing him into exile, because it has taught him the value of compassion. (Given that the Tibetan diaspora has enriched the West with an unprecedented influx of gifted teachers willing to share their mystical knowledge, we should be grateful as well.) The Dalai Lama has never said that China was justified in what it did, and he has never stopped fighting passionately for the liberation of Tibet from Communist rule. The two attitudes—gratefulness and the struggle against injustice—are not mutually exclusive.

Working with Symbolic sight is one of the greatest skills we can develop, because it gives us "perceptual leverage." We enter a more detached state of consciousness, interpreting the events in our lives as spiritual challenges that are meant to enhance our growth. This is especially true of illness, as we will see in Chapter 6. Even though so many of life's lessons are enormously painful, at their core they are nonetheless positive. The capacity to view a crisis irrespective of its physical details requires acceptance of the events and a willingness to "take up your bed and walk." Once you begin walking again, particularly through the Symbolic realm, you will become positioned for healing and will never again return to using ordinary perceptual skills.

Under the influence of Aquarian energy, then, we will construct an entirely new model of health. We will expand it beyond its Piscean definition as "the absence of physical illness" and realize that health includes our thoughts, occupation, relationships, philosophy of life, spiritual practices, and much more. The Aquarian model does not measure health solely by the level at which our physical body functions; our management of our entire energy system becomes another criterion. From that perspective, one can be physically limited but very healthy, like the actor Christopher Reeve, who in the acceptance of his physical tragedy has been able to release his spirit as a source of inspiration to so many.

In line with Aquarian holism, we have come to see that we are not the only form of conscious life on this planet. In ways we may not yet fully understand, we are energetically linked to every other form of life, whether animal, insect, plant, or microbe. As our research into the realm of energy expands, we will discover that our personal health is influenced by the vibrational patterns of our entire global society and environment. Unfortunately, we long ago passed up our chance to take the "wisdom path" in dealing with environmental dilemmas. We are now destined, as a global community, to take the "woe path," on which we will be forced to change many of our habits to avoid global environmental, economic, and health-related disasters.

From a Symbolic perspective, however, these crises and the changes we may be forced to make will also mark the closure of the Piscean parent-child pattern and the emergence of the Aquarian partnership pattern. We are witnessing the end of the dependence of the individual on government, typified by our rethinking of the American welfare system along with Social Security and medical entitlements programs. We have even begun to see the first hopeful signs that the Piscean fascination with chemical medicine—which produced the myth that science holds the keys to all physical mysteries—is coming to an end. In its place is emerging an Aquarian model that views health and healing as a lifestyle in which treatment for illness includes every part of life.

At the same time, however, some misleading Aquarian myths regarding health are being introduced, among them the belief that illness can be healed by the power of the mind alone and that a tranquil spirit can stop the aging process. The mind alone, without the aid of the human spirit and emotions, is limited in its influence on the body. And although the unity of body, mind, and spirit can indeed retard the deterioration of the physical body, we have yet to prove that we can prevent drastic changes in our physical appearance or its ultimate disintegration.

In isolating these astrological ages of Aries, Pisces, and Aquarius and identifying each with an expansion of the scope of human consciousness, it's easy to misconstrue the progression of human growth as strictly linear. Truth—especially spiritual truth—is rarely so simple, of course. In some ways, the ages have a cyclical quality that makes their progression resemble a spiral more closely than a straight line. The global unity of the Aquarian age, for instance, mirrors the tribal unity of the Arien age, but with much more positive consequences. And both of these eras may reflect the unity of the fabled Golden Age of Goddess culture, when civilization worshiped essentially one feminine divinity under many manifestations, when neither sex was dominant, and when the prevailing mode of social interaction was partnership and cooperation. For reasons that remain unclear, this seemingly idyllic culture was not intended to survive as it was. Perhaps humanity had to progress through cycles of creation, destruction, and re-creation similar to those of Hindu cosmology to get where we are today.

To be sure, mistakes have been made along the way, but there is no mistake in the overall pattern of our development. We are here for a reason, and it is up to us to learn from our collective past. One thing we will certainly need to learn is how to recognize and work with Individual and Symbolic power, and to become fluent in the language of energy—to speak chakras, as I put it. At the same time, we must be able to integrate the three forms of power—Tribal, Individual, and Symbolic—that have evolved during the Arien, Piscean, and Aquarian ages, because they are all at work in us simultaneously. In the next chapter, we will begin discussing the shift from Tribal to Individual and ultimately Symbolic power, and identifying some of the signs by which you can recognize this transformation in yourself.

Chapter Four

✦

BEGINNING THE JOURNEY
TO INDIVIDUAL
AND SYMBOLIC POWER

We all begin our lives saturated in Tribal or group belief patterns, starting with those of our biological tribes. Tribal beliefs, by their very nature, are held by the group; some are universally recognized as truth, such as that murder is wrong, while others are unique to a particular group, such as the belief that "ours is the only true religion." Even before we reach the age of reason (around seven), our energy circuits have been connected to Tribal belief patterns through the influence of our Tribal elders (parents, teachers, religious, and political leaders), beginning with the belief patterns that are aligned to our first chakra, and then continuing with those inherent in our second and third chakras. By the time we are four years old, all three chakras are fully active. (Later in life, as we develop our Individual power, the fourth, fifth, and sixth chakras become activated in turn. The seventh chakra kicks in when we learn to see the events of our life through Symbolic sight, recognizing the archetypal patterns that underlie many of our own actions.)

We begin to emerge from the Tribal mindset and into Individual (and eventually Symbolic) power when we begin to pursue questions about how we relate to the rest of the universe: "What about me? How do I fit my needs into the obligations I have? In fact, what *are* my needs?" This process begins subtly, the same way that you might begin to lose interest in a hobby or a certain type of food and become fascinated with other pastimes and cuisines. Of course, a shift in perception about your place in the world is far more serious than dropping a hobby. Moving away from your accustomed views of life and everything that your life includes can be a troublesome, fearful process.

It may help you to realize that moving from the Tribal mind-set into Individual power is inevitable. Most of us will arrive at some point in our lives when the world with which we are most familiar no longer works for us. For some people, it happens more than once. We are meant to outgrow ourselves; indeed, we can no more avoid this development than we can stop the aging process. The only question is how gracefully—and healthily—we will handle the transition. Sometimes the catalyst is an emotional or inner crisis, and sometimes it is a simple life choice that ultimately leads us in a direction we didn't anticipate. Inevitably, each of us will reach the moment when the place where we have felt most comfortable becomes so *un*comfortable that we feel as if we are suffocating in the stale air of our own history.

Self-exploration is an important, rewarding component of spiritual growth. Yet the opportunity to know ourselves often scares us because, as we saw with the second myth about healing, we associate the pursuit of self-knowledge with grueling loneliness. We are Tribal by design, of course, but we are meant to learn that *all* of life is an extension of our Tribe, not only those people related to us genetically or those closest to us through friendship or acquaintanceship.

Consciousness means becoming aware that we are all a part of one thriving energy system. We learn this by getting to know ourselves apart from familiar circumstances that allow us the safety of illusions, such as believing that someone will always be around to take care of us and to make our decisions for us. Living with such beliefs prevents us from discovering the content of our own minds and hearts, so we are usually not permitted to live through another's mind for long. Conversely, we are not usually permitted to interfere indefinitely in another person's needs and right to journey inward, to separate and individuate, whether that person is a spouse, child, or friend.

We are meant to learn about the power of our thoughts and feelings and thereby to discover the greater degree of choice that is inherent in their power. Choice is born out of opposing polarities—the twin fish of Pisces. It activates our experiences, individual and spiritual, and expresses our beliefs. We can choose to be kind or cruel, forgiving or vengeful, generous or miserly, compassionate or judgmental. Choices like these take on far greater significance as we realize that their consequences reach far beyond ourselves and our intimates, and that those consequences play out within our biology. Every choice we make, spoken or unspoken, influences the atmosphere of the room where we stand or the home we have just entered or left. For all we know, our choices may even influence weather patterns. Western culture has only begun to take seriously the power of choice that Hindu and Buddhist practices have taught as right thought, right speech, right action.

Consciousness is about coming to terms with our Individual power, with the power of our thoughts and actions to have widespread effects. As long as we remain in the sway of Tribal power, our ability to choose and our capacity to grow in self-responsibility are limited. Within the Tribal mind, we are often unaware of the complex of psychological and emotional forces that acts on our decision-making processes. We tend to make decisions by reaction or habit. But as we begin to explore ourselves, we gradually expand the way we define ourselves and our role in life. As we take responsibility for our external actions, as well as for our thoughts and attitudes, we begin to see our energy connections to others and to the vital life-force itself.

For the sake of our personal evolution, we need to extricate ourselves from the grip of Tribal power, to break down and break through our psyches and to come into contact with our shadow side. The polarities of Pisces and of Individual power symbolize that there is no simple answer to anything, that every virtue has its shadow. As the Lord said to the prophet Isaiah near the end of the age of Aries, "I form the light and I create the darkness; I make well-being and I create disaster; I, Yahveh, do all these things" (Isaiah 45:7). By the same token, every decision to act eliminates the possibility of another kind of action, yet we need to accept the fact that there may often be no ideal decision. What matters most is not the choice itself but the *reason* behind the choice. If we choose something out of fear, the result of our action may be unsatisfactory and unstable; if we choose in faith, the outcome of our action will probably take us in the direction we need to go, however haltingly.

Our lives change externally as we change internally. One follows the other naturally, and try as we will, we cannot stop this dynamic. As is often the case, we will try desperately to take with us those people about whom we care most, or to hold steady the external components of our lives, even as our internal fires rage and threaten to consume us. We will try to describe to our family and friends what we are experiencing and hope that they will relate to it in some way, or perhaps they will find the landscape we are exploring within ourselves attractive enough to jump into the world behind their own eyes. Sometimes we succeed; often we do not. Our choice to proceed on the journey must be made in faith and cannot be dependent on who chooses to come along with us. As psychologist and theologian Sam Keen is fond of saying, two of the most important questions for your life journey are "Where am I going?" and "Who will go with me?" And it is very important to ask them of yourself *in that order.*

It helps to keep in mind that the instinct of the tribe is to discourage its members from venturing too far from the familiar. More often than not, when you are on the journey toward self-discovery, you will be met with opposition. You would be making a mistake to take this response personally; it should be viewed as an act of Tribal love, or at least Tribal loyalty, because tribes, by design, strive to keep their numbers together.

But your desire to have your experience noted and validated may well be one that friends and family members cannot satisfy, because they are not experiencing what you are going through. They may have trouble understanding your isolation, when they are still surrounded by those they love; they have no need to penetrate into the deeper meaning of their own lives when they are happy living at the surface. Many of us initially shy away from the search because we know intuitively that it likely will lead to life changes. In fact, I doubt that those of us on the search would make as much progress as we do if we knew ahead of time the full extent of the difficulties we will face.

Your journey of self-discovery may have begun without your even knowing it. The signs that it has are not difficult to see, once you know what you're looking for. Here are some of the most common and telling ones.

The Signals That Self-Discovery Has Begun

+ A growing discomfort with your familiar environment, which can manifest as feelings that you are no longer satisfied with your occupation or even with your primary relationship.

+ The inability to identify why you are saturated with depression or exhaustion.

+ A penetrating sensation of loneliness, often accompanied by anxiety that your isolation will never end.

+ An absolute awareness that something in your life has changed and that, although you may not be certain what the future holds, you definitely cannot turn back and live as you had before.

+ A growing curiosity about your personal needs and a passion to discover what they are and to have them validated by someone who understands what you are experiencing.

The deep feelings of loneliness that can accompany an awakening require some level of validation, particularly if you are not surrounded by people who understand what you are experiencing. (If this is your situation, seeking out the company of a consciousness support group or attending workshops on related themes can be extremely useful and grounding.)

✦ The emergence of skills you never knew you possessed, such as the ability to heal or counsel others, and a shift in your perception of reality. This frequently includes a heightened sensitivity to energetic or vibrational patterns transmitted by people and environments. You shift from relating to the external world through your five senses to awakening your multisensory and intuitive abilities. Even though survival intuition, or gut instinct, is always active in everyone, this new sensitivity reflects the emergence of a much deeper intuitive skill. It can develop into the kinds of sensitivity one needs for healing with, say, Therapeutic Touch or acupuncture, or it may simply assist you in becoming a more insightful individual.

✦ A shift in your relationship to time. Within Tribal power, time is an external linear force that moves you through the stages of your life from youth to elder years. What you accomplish and how rapidly you succeed are calibrated to Tribal speed. If the tribe believes it takes a year of treatment and five years of good health to be considered clear of cancer, then that is the timing that a Tribal believer will expect. Within Individual power, however, time becomes increasingly relative, as you discover the power of your conscious mind. You no longer need to be controlled by group timing; instead, you have the option of pursuing how self-empowerment and the healing of your internal self can influence the speed of recovery of your physical body. This sense of timing extends to the speed at which you can create something new for yourself. Rather than thinking, "I'm too old to start again," you can believe that age has nothing to do with creativity, love, or the enjoyment of life.

+ An increase in sensitivities to certain foods, fabrics, environmental toxins, and medications such as aspirin and common cold remedies. You may develop allergies to substances that previously did not affect your system, such as wheat, dairy products, and caffeine.

+ A growing curiosity about areas related to self-development, either by choice or necessity.

+ An emerging sense of a new identity, which can include discovering new ambitions or desiring to live an entirely new lifestyle. You may choose to leave city life for the country, or to take a pay cut in exchange for more free time and a chance to pursue other interests.

+ Sensations of liberation unlike any you have ever known before, as if you have broken away from invisible chains that had attached you to repetitive patterns of behavior that no longer suit the size of your spirit.

+ A need for more contact with nature or more time alone.

+ A growing dissatisfaction with institutional religion and a need to seek out spirituality. You may also begin to have spiritual experiences, such as deep states of meditation, a call to a new path in life, or even a Kundalini awakening.

+ Endless boredom and a loss of appetite for everything that once brought you satisfaction and contentment.

+ The development of an illness that cannot be successfully treated by allopathic medical procedures.

Everyone on the path to Individual power will become familiar with at least one of these signals or stages, and some may experience several or even all of them. Each one represents a kind of challenge: either a new irritation or discomfort that we need to alleviate, or a new orientation, skill, or power that we may want to utilize. Enduring and resolving challenges seems to be the hall-mark of the journey, often described as the desert experience or the dark night of the soul. This dark night of our soul's emergence may seem daunting and discouraging, but growing into Individual power inevitably creates some pain and discomfort. Yet it also offers us the chance to emerge at a higher level of mastery and satisfaction. Like moving into a new home, starting a new job, or entering a new relationship, the difficulties we face in embarking on the journey often mask its potential for greater joy and fulfillment.

Let's take a look at some of the forms that the challenge to our old Tribal patterns of living can take, and how we can go about transforming them into new beginnings.

ILLNESS AS TRANSFORMATIVE VEHICLE

Disease is one of the most frequent eye-openers on the journey toward consciousness and self-discovery. Disease demands immediate attention and cannot be ignored. When our wake-up call takes the shape of a life-threatening illness, we are not given the option to ignore it. Disease can be the means through which we encounter the power of our psyche and spirit.

As we have already seen in Chapter 2, negativity is not always the root cause of illness. Sometimes illness is the result of genetic or environmental factors over which we seem to have little control. As difficult as it may be to consider, illness is also sometimes the answer to prayer, because it can be the means through which we discover our most valuable abilities and contribute the most to others. Such an illness can be thought of as a turning point at which you must exercise your power to choose. Faced with a crisis that demands resolution through a shift in consciousness and lifestyle, you need to search for the potential for spiritual growth inherent in the situation. To avoid developing a negative attitude toward your illness, think of it as an invitation to discover a higher level of consciousness. The recent medical literature is filled with stories of people who responded to a heart attack or cancer by changing their diet and taking up exercise along with some kind of stress-reduction program that incorporated yoga and meditation—and who discovered a genuine affinity for these practices. As a result, many changed their lives dramatically, walking through the doorway opened by life-threatening illness into a life of spiritual rebirth.

I believe that all illnesses can be thought of as transformation experiences, because illness demands that we pay attention to the healing process, which alone contains the possibility of change. When illness develops because of a negative behavior pattern—substance abuse, smoking, high stress levels, a stultifying job or relationship—personal change becomes part of the healing process. At the same time, looking upon an illness as an opportunity to grow in self-awareness activates the potential for healing that lies dormant when you take a passive position or descend into self-pity. As I point out to people in my workshops, "Verbs heal, nouns don't."

WHEN THE CHALLENGE IS DISEASE

At age 41, Ann was married, the mother of four, and actively involved in her community when, surprisingly, she was diagnosed with lupus. She had absolutely no familiarity with alternative medicine, and so she naturally turned to conventional medicine for treatment. She was given steroids to take on a frequent basis, and her weight skyrocketed by almost 70 pounds over her normal body weight, which had been around 135 pounds.

Ann's physician informed her that lupus was an illness for which there was essentially no cure. The best that she could hope for was to achieve a state of remission through drug therapy. Ann felt that she had no choice but to accept this prognosis and treatment plan, but as the months of chemical infusion continued, she became extremely depressed and physically exhausted. She suffered from continual feelings of guilt about being unable to attend to the needs of her family, leaning more and more on her 16-year-old daughter to help with the preparation of meals, shopping, and housekeeping. Her daughter, trying her best to help out, soon showed signs of resentment, since her social life was cut in half and she was hardly prepared to handle many of her new responsibilities.

The tension in the household finally became so extreme that Ann's husband suggested that she seek therapeutic help. It took Ann another couple of months before she responded to that suggestion, but when she did, she met a therapist who happened to be actively involved in the alternative healing community and who helped her learn about other treatments available for lupus, from acupuncture to visualization to aromatherapy.

At the same time, Ann was learning about herself. Her therapist made it clear that she could not approach these treatments with the same attitude with which she had approached drug therapy. "Drugs work regardless of your state of mind," she said, "but that's not true for alternative treatments. Those rely on your conscious participation; in fact, the more conscious you are, the more effectively they work." Inspired by that knowledge, Ann worked to educate herself through books, tapes, and meetings with a support group.

Through this journey, Ann made several remarkable transitions. The most dramatic was her discovery of the difference between the support she received through her religion and the support she was finding through other spiritual practices. When she had first learned of her diagnosis, Ann had felt that she was being punished for something. As she grew to have a more intimate relationship with God through her new practices, she was able to consider God in very different terms and to view her illness from an entirely new perspective.

"The first thing I discovered," Ann said, "was that the deep guilt that I had been carrying with me since the diagnosis—guilt about my no longer being able to be the wife and mother that I had been before—actually stemmed from my belief that I was somehow a bad person. I was ashamed for having become ill and I assumed that my family must feel the same way about me.

"As I learned to approach God from a point of view that was not tied to a specific religion, but that was more generally spiritual," she continued, "I was introduced to the possibility that illness is sometimes the means through which God leads us to discover more about ourselves. It had never occurred to me, for example, that I had a kind of power within me that was enhanced by positive thought. I mean, I had always assumed that it was better to be an optimistic person than a complainer, but I had never really connected that notion to having the power to strengthen my spirit in such a way that it could positively enhance my health. And because I had grown up with the notion that God randomly sent blessings or challenges, the view that nothing is random and nothing is really a punishment felt like the deepest form of liberation I had ever experienced. This kind of spirituality gave me hope—and not just the hope that said if I prayed enough, maybe God would hear my prayers. Instead, I began to believe that God hears every prayer and that healing is not necessarily a matter of receiving a physical cure. It may mean that you discover, as I did, that you have a great deal more courage in you than you ever knew about.

"I realized that although I would love to heal lupus permanently from my body, I also wanted to heal the many insecurities that had caused me to live such a sheltered life. All the while I thought I was safe, I was actually a frightened person afraid to try anything new. I am healing that part of myself, and feeling better about who I am than I ever thought was possible. I no longer feel controlled by all the 'what ifs' that used to torment me. I may still have lupus, but I am healthier in many ways than before I had this illness. Now I have hope that if I keep on this path, I can and eventually will heal at the physical level as well."

In time, Ann's illness went into remission, and although no one can predict how long that state will last, she remains hopeful that should the illness reactivate, she will be prepared to confront her situation with courage.

WHEN THE CHALLENGE IS FEAR OF AGING

You don't always need a life-threatening disease or debilitating illness to get you started on your personal journey. A man named Jacques, whom I met a few years ago in a workshop, told the most delightful story of what got him moving. He was an extremely successful businessman who had given himself every possible treat that money could buy. He had traveled to unusual places, owned three homes—one in the French Alps—mingled with interesting friends, and just generally enjoyed a great life. On his fortieth birthday, as he was pondering what special present to buy for himself, he took a long look at himself in the mirror. He noticed that he was completely out of shape physically, right down to the "love handles" on his hips, so he decided that rather than give himself a lavish conventional present, he would take up jogging and spend the next year getting himself in shape. He admitted that on that first day he was far more inspired by the fear of aging than by any higher motive, but nonetheless, on his birthday, he went out for his first run. After only three blocks he pulled up, coughing, wheezing, and out of breath. He realized that if he was going to succeed at his jogging commitment, he would have to quit smoking. By eight o'clock that night, he was an ex-smoker.

Within four months, Jacques's newfound dedication to improving his health led him to develop an interest in nutrition— an area about which he had had little concern prior to his fortieth birthday. He read up on various nutritional programs and eventually decided to give up his heavily fat-filled diet, limit his intake of red meat, and eat mainly fresh fruit and vegetables.

By the time his forty-first birthday arrived, Jacques was a picture of health. Just as significantly, his interest in health had made him curious about other factors that might influence health:

mental attitude, belief patterns, and personal needs. He began to review his life or, as he put it, to discover his inner self. When he had been focused solely on business, he had had absolutely no awareness that anything else—much less any*one* else—mattered all that much. His contentment had led to complacency. But since beginning his sojourn into himself, he couldn't help but think about what was going on with all the people with whom he was in contact on a regular basis.

One day Jacques got the idea to invite a group of his close friends and business associates over to his home for an evening of self-exploration. Naturally, he told me with glee, he waited until they had arrived before he told them why he had asked them to come. They were expecting Jacques to introduce them to a new business venture in which they could join; when he told them what his real motive was, they clearly wanted to fly out of the room. "But because I was the richest man in the room," Jacques added while laughing with delight at his scheme, "they had to stay."

He opened the evening by describing his own process of transformation, adding that whether or not any of them realized it, they too were frozen in an endless cycle of blind achievement, waiting to wake up. He would like them to explore waking up. One by one these men began speaking about themselves in a new way— exploring their feelings about their occupations, their lifestyles, their families. Although it was awkward for them at first, their discomfort gradually vanished. They ended the evening by promising to meet again within the month for another such experience.

Within six months, the men were meeting on a regular basis and had actually expanded the group. Their discussions eventually took them out of themselves and into areas related to spirituality, global crises, and what they could do for the world that had given them so much. They each pledged to work for the betterment of the planet. Their gatherings by now had turned into a mixture of personal sharings and a kind of think tank, in which they came up with people or projects that could benefit from their support.

Jacques's journey is an especially rich story, partly because he had at first appeared to be a fully developed individual. At the time of his awakening, he was self-motivated, self-determined, self-confident, and highly accomplished, and so he hardly seemed like someone who needed to get in touch with himself. But "individual" as defined by the Tribal mind and "Individual" as understood within the context of the evolution of consciousness have two entirely different meanings.

An "individual," according to the Tribal mind, is little more than an amalgam of one's physical identity and the strength of one's ego, which here means the part of the self that we know through external experiences, combined with our feelings about our physical appearance. But as a level of consciousness, "Individual" refers to the part of ourselves that is transphysical, embodying inner characteristics that come from spiritual growth and that give us stamina and power independent of group approval.

WHEN YOUR LIFE NO LONGER SUITS YOU

Although Jacques's journey of self-discovery began almost whimsically, most people begin the journey as the result of some serious life crisis. During one workshop, Simon, an attorney, recounted his experience. Simon had become a lawyer because his father was a judge and had told him that, from the time Simon was a small child, his dream had been for them to have a father-and-son law practice. So strongly influenced had he been by his father's ambitions for him, Simon admitted, that he did not realize until he was into his early thirties that he might be allowed to have ambitions of his own.

Simon became a lawyer right on schedule, as he put it, and had begun a law practice by the time he was 26. He was married at 27 and became a father at 29. He was, of course, expected to rear his daughter to become a lawyer. In fact, Simon's father remarked upon her birth that while he hadn't expected his son's firstborn to be a girl, she nevertheless might still do fine as an attorney.

By the time Simon was 34, he was on the verge of a nervous breakdown. He could no longer relate to his wife, either verbally or sexually, and he could no longer handle the responsibilities of his job. The only support he received from his family was their suggestion that he take a longer vacation. One day, as Simon was staring out the window of his office, his secretary came in and made a remark that caught him completely off guard. "You need therapy," she said. "Do you know that?"

At first, Simon found her remark insulting and told her so. She said that she hadn't intended to be insulting; rather, she had noticed the gradual decline in his spirits and demeanor and suspected that the pressure of his life was becoming greater than he knew how to manage. A therapist, she told him, is not a person to whom crazy people go for help. It's someone sane people seek out when they realize that everything *around* them has gone crazy.

Simon admitted that he didn't know any therapists, so his secretary suggested that he go to hers. She picked up his phone, dialed her therapist, and arranged an appointment for the following week. Simon made her promise that she would not breathe a word of this to anyone. When the day of the appointment came, he slipped out of the office, made his way to the therapist's office, and spent his first visit repeating that he had no idea why he was there or what he was supposed to do.

The therapist began by asking Simon about his life, his family, and his occupation. Then she asked him the one question he had never even considered asking himself: "What did you want for your own life?"

"To become a lawyer, get married, have a family," he replied. "Exactly what I have."

"Oh, really? Then why are you so 'content' right now?" she asked in a challenging tone of voice. "Have you ever considered that maybe that's not what you wanted?"

Simon told her that he had never given that thought a moment's consideration. "But what if you were to think about that now?" she asked.

"Oh, I couldn't do that," he answered. "What good would it do anyway? All my choices have been made."

The therapist suggested that they meet again the following week and that between now and then he spend some time pondering what choices he might have made, or would like to make, or would be almost afraid even to consider. Simon didn't want to do his assignment, but the questions had already been implanted and so, like it or not, he had begun the journey into himself.

During the next week, Simon found it almost impossible to sleep at night. His thoughts returned to his childhood, and to all the plans and expectations that had been predetermined for him. He began to experience rage such as he had never known before. Afraid of what he might say to his father—or of holding in what he would *like* to say—Simon avoided communication with him altogether.

Simon's wife noticed the obvious increase in his anxiety, but he was unable to confide in her that he had begun therapy, because he believed she would panic at the very notion. At his next appointment all he could do was tell his therapist that he had no idea what he wanted for his life because he had never before been given the opportunity to consider that question. All he had come to realize during the past week, he said, was that he had never been given freedom of choice in any area of his life—from what he would do for a living to whom he would marry. In other words, he had lived completely within the Tribal mind.

"I told my therapist that I loved my wife," Simon added, "but I kept to myself the horrible realization that I had come to, which was that I wasn't in love with her at all."

As the weeks continued, Simon was guided step by step into the journey of self-discovery. He found the first stages to be the most liberating thing he had ever done for himself—and the most frightening. Eventually he realized that he no longer had the heart to do any of the things he was doing. He wanted to take time to explore everything he had missed along the way. Finally the day came when he told his family that he indeed wanted a vacation, but not just from the business. He announced that he needed time to rethink every choice that had ever been made for him, to see if that was really what he wanted for himself.

In the end, Simon continued working as an attorney, but he changed from corporate to private practice. And in the course of these changes, he met another woman with whom he fell in love, one who was open to the rich internal territory that he continued to explore passionately with the help of his therapist. He was not surprised when his parents, who had not supported his new choices, did not accept his decision to divorce his wife either. Simon concluded his account to the workshop this way: "I remain hopeful that one day my family will know me as I am now coming to know myself. I am sad about the distance between us, but at the same time I am finally content."

Simon's story is a classic example of separation from Tribal influence by birthing the Individual within. In the midst of our own lives, we subtly begin feeling out of place. The people and places with which we are most familiar no longer generate the energy we need to thrive. A state of depression is triggered, but we can't figure out why, especially if nothing obvious in our lives has changed.

At a deeper level, of course, we know exactly what is occurring and why it frightens us. We are not born devoid of knowledge about the working power of our spiritual nature; quite the contrary, we know instinctively that every internal change we make, every shift in perspective or belief, automatically activates an external shift in our lives. Try as we may, we cannot stop that shift—which should be encouraging if we are trying to heal an illness.

Simon's initial fear of evaluating himself had been activated by the realization that something had begun to awaken inside him that would ultimately cause his life to change. Change scares us so much that many people will unconsciously sabotage their own healing process rather than make changes in their emotional and psychological lives that will affect a shift in their biology. Change the emotion, change your energy, and you change your biology. As I am fond of saying, your biography becomes your biology. Although there are no guarantees about healing, if you are able to enter into a process of change, then you maximize your chances of healing.

THE POWER OF THE AWAKENED SELF

Once you have made the transition to Individual power, once you have opened yourself to this form of energy, you soon learn that self-discovery is not a process that ends. On the contrary, self-expression and self-care become the rule rather than the exception. Individual power has its own set of priorities, its own vocabulary, its own values. You may feel as if you encounter more challenges than you have ever experienced before. This is because you have unlocked a potential in yourself that had previously been asleep, and you discover that you have abilities, perceptions, and other energy tools that you had not allowed yourself to own earlier.

You have, for example, permission to investigate and state your personal needs. Although the skill of self-expression is often exceedingly difficult to get the hang of, you can reach out for support to learn it. Fueled by Individual power, you come to understand personal boundaries and what it means to protect yourself from influences that don't support your growth. You begin to understand the need to love and provide for yourself. I don't meet many people who can recall having learned as a child that they must first love themselves in order to love another person fully and unselfishly, though I do meet many who recall with great delight that they certainly were loved as children. More often,

I encounter people who were well into the mid-years before they felt comfortable even coming close to the notion of loving themselves.

Self-love is a relatively new and much misunderstood concept, despite the fact that it is the most obvious corollary of Christ's commandment to love your neighbor *as yourself.* Of course, self-love can be problematical: In its initial stages, it may manifest in episodes of self-indulgence and narcissism. But these episodes may actually be beneficial, because they challenge us to introduce personal boundaries where, until now, we may not have defined any. But following the self-indulgent stage comes a genuine need to explore our own emotional needs.

At its best, self-love is the capacity to take care of ourselves, to make choices within our present lifestyle that nurture us and renew our vitality. For some of us, that may mean maintaining a steady exercise routine, while for others it may mean taking off for the country every so often. Still others need the regular healing touch of a massage treatment, a monthly facial, or something more social. You may require the company of an entirely new social group—for instance, people who are dedicated to maintaining the environment, living organically, or maintaining a spiritual practice of some kind. Or you may find that you need the freedom to live alone and to get to know yourself apart from ordinary social pressures. In some cases you may express your self-love by making a vow never again to allow abuse to come into your life.

Regardless of what needs surface as you learn to know and love yourself, the important point is to give yourself the right of choice, self-expression, and self-respect. In this way, you will discover firsthand the truth that not until you can love yourself can you love another.

Perhaps the most significant aspect of opening yourself to Individual power that is that your new atmosphere of healing provides you with an entirely new profile of what it means to be a healthy person. Beyond the old inaccurate definition that a healthy person is someone who has no physical illness, your health becomes first and foremost determined by your consciousness. Even for those of you who are actually suffering from a physical illness, particularly one that is painful, your belief in the lessons and meaning inherent in your illness can generate a sustaining hope and energy.

Our spiritual needs must be met if our bodies are to thrive. This realization has become a fundamental part of the processes of maintaining health and healing. We have also opened ourselves to the possibility, if not probability, that we may have lived before and that those previous lifetimes are filtering influences into this lifetime, including influences on our health. Our knowledge of nutrition and food supplements, combined with our knowledge of healing techniques both from Eastern cultures and from within our own holistic culture, have made available to us healing possibilities that challenge the familiar prognoses of allopathic medicine.

All of these factors give us great advantages and extraordinary options, should we need them for our personal healing. Ultimately, everything we learn about our deeper selves enhances not only our health but also the quality of our physical life as such. The goal is to embrace fully and enjoy our life in our bodies as consciously as possible.

MOVING INTO SYMBOLIC POWER

Symbolic power is by far the most potent level of insight available to us. Making contact with the archetypal realm allows us to see beyond the physical meaning of events and view them as Divine opportunities to evolve our consciousness. Symbolic sight perceives a dimension that mystics have described as more real than the physical, more powerful than the tangible.

Symbolic consciousness encounters the Divine mind with less interference than Individual consciousness. It perceives the higher vibratory level known as eternity and can manifest as a rich, internal sensation, a spiritual encounter, or some kind of psychic experience. It can also take the form of a deeply personal relationship with nature, a creative expression, or an extraordinarily creative insight, breakthrough, or solution.

A Sample of Symbolic Reasoning

In Chapter 6, I will give you a detailed, step-by-step guide for applying these three forms of power to every crisis and issue in your life, not just physical illness. For now, however, I would just like to give you a sense of where you are going, a brief taste of the strength and beauty of the Symbolic mind.

Suppose you have just been diagnosed with a serious condition, perhaps cancer or multiple sclerosis. Both illnesses have frightening prognoses. Upon receiving such a diagnosis, most people experience shock and maybe anger, a natural response. Eventually, however, you have to respond to the news by undertaking an external treatment program, so you begin to take medications. To accommodate your healing, you may also change your nutritional program.

As the weeks pass and you do not receive the results you had hoped for, a voice inside of you begins to ask, "Why did this have to happen to me? And why now, just when things were beginning to go well?" Or perhaps the voice asks, "Why should I be surprised that this happened to me? Bad things always happen to me. I should be used to this by now, and I certainly shouldn't expect a miracle."

Depression sets in. People around you try in every way they know to offer you hope, but you can no longer make the connection that hope is anywhere to be found in your universe.

Then you meet a person who offers you a new way of interpreting your situation. Imagine, you are told, that every one of us carries within us a part that feels like a Victim. For some of us, our

Victim surfaces whenever we are in an intimate relationship. For others, our Victim begins to speak every time we are asked for our opinion on something. For still others, our Victim is forever telling us ahead of time what to expect when we get "there," no matter where "there" is.

You comment to your new adviser that you can relate to that and that you know people who fit every one of those descriptions, yourself included.

"That's right," you are told. "Everyone carries a Victim within, and because of that, no one should take their Victim personally. It's simply a part of the natural makeup of the human psyche." Now you are asked, "What if you were given the opportunity to face that part of yourself and rid yourself of that negative influence once and for all. Would you take it?"

You ponder for a moment, then respond that you would. Then you are told that the release would have to be of an experiential nature. You will have to meet your Victim face to face, to encounter the Victim in a circumstance in which he or she is most powerful so that you can discover the part of yourself that is capable of challenging this force. You agree.

Then an illness develops within your body. Now is your opportunity, and you ask, "How do I meet the Victim in me?"

"Does this illness make you feel like a Victim?" you're asked.

"Yes, it makes me feel helpless, contaminated, defeated, and betrayed by my body. It makes me feel afraid."

"Then let's focus on those feelings," you are instructed, "and not on the illness. Be guided by this truth: Do not take your challenge personally, regardless of whether it is an illness, a relationship trauma, or a job crisis. The first step is not to separate yourself from the challenge but to face clearly the fears and feelings of being a Victim that the crisis activates in you. The second step is to walk directly into those feelings. The illness is not the issue, and you must repeat this to yourself a hundred or a thousand times a day if necessary. The issue is the loss of power that the illness generates in you.

"Then go on a quest to find those things that make you feel powerful. Make decisions that will bring power into your system. Develop an idea of faith and what you can do to put yourself in closer contact with the spirit within you. Repeat to yourself again that the illness is not the issue. You are facing the part of yourself that has always made you feel defeated and frightened, and the illness is merely the means to confront that bugaboo in earnest.

"Then dwell on your strength. Celebrate each accomplishment you make daily, regardless of whether you think the accomplishment is big or small. Symbolically, every accomplishment is big. Look for the patterns of strength and weakness that have always influenced you. Invite the patterns of weakness to show themselves, one a day if necessary, so that you can choose alternatives—and then make those choices.

"Each day, the Victim in you will become weaker and the Victor will become stronger. Each day, you will feel a deeper connection to life, a life you feel in charge of rather than a life that has taken charge of you. This is the way you were meant to live because it makes you want to live—empowerment makes you feel that you can create anything.

"And then one day you notice that you are not conscious of the Victim any longer. You have the strength to face anything that you need to face, whether it's the creation of a new life or the release of a life lived fully at the end. This is the way we were meant to know ourselves, in a deeply personal way while recognizing the universally impersonal nature of our experiences."

Archetypal reasoning, such as you have just sampled, is the most richly liberating form of sight that you can develop within yourself. Combined with your Tribal and Individual power, the Symbolic mind gives you the ability to interpret the negative challenges of your life and realize that each one is a positive gift, even if that gift is not immediately evident.

Symbolic sight is transcendent of time. It is eternal sight, containing all the truth ever acquired within the human experience. When you utilize it, you are free to tap into the teachings of the great spiritual and philosophical masters of every generation and every culture and see no barrier to their application today. You have the liberty to recognize that today's crises are connected to events yet to unfold, and to events that have already occurred, realizing that the response you give in this present moment affects both the past and the future.

The Symbolic mind is a fountain of strength and truth, and those who have made contact with it are capable of surviving anything. They are also capable of experiencing a resurrection that remains purely mythical to those who cannot grasp that the power of the Symbolic or unseen dimension of life.

Symbolic power is inherent in each of us. It is the essence of the eighth chakra, the power center that resonates above our physical body. Half personal, half impersonal, it is forever trying to seduce us into entering and discovering our true energy and nature. It is our unconscious self, the part that longs to come out into the open and become a conscious ally, not drawing us away from rapture-filled contact with physical life, but giving us the freedom to embrace all that life is without fear that we are not powerful enough to know life fully.

RECEIVING GUIDANCE

In every situation, no matter how challenging, you have the option to pursue the meaning behind the event. In some cases, this may simply mean trusting that there must ultimately be a positive reason for what has happened, and that when and if the time becomes appropriate, the meaning will be revealed. This is hardly an easy response to have in a crisis, especially during the life-and-death situation that illness can often be. But it is the response that will bring you the most power and the clearest guidance.

We respond to crises using the three powers in the same order as we have developed them, both historically and individually: Tribal, Individual, and Symbolic. This response is automatic; it is the way we are programmed to handle situations. Our initial response to the diagnosis of an illness, for instance, is somewhat like our response to an earthquake. The world beneath our feet is shaken to the core—something powerful and unexpected has happened that can potentially change the most important parts of our lives, including our most intimate relationships and our occupational security. It is almost impossible to have a positive reaction right away, or to see hope immediately coming over the horizon. And so we react to illness first at the Tribal level, because we need to get a grip on the physical implications of something so potentially threatening. We need to understand the complexities of the disease and the options for treatment, and we have to organize our lives so as to cope with the illness.

After the crisis of illness penetrates our Tribal mind through the lower chakras, it filters up to our Individual mind. This is a crucial and terrifying shift because as long as we keep thinking and acting within the Tribal mind, our experience will be absorbed and supported by the group. But when it enters our Individual mind, activating our psychological and emotional reactions, we are on our own. No one else can silence the fear that speaks to us at night as we lie in bed contemplating what we must face tomorrow.

Yet in the midst of this frightening journey comes the opportunity to move beyond despair and seek an inner dialogue from which can emerge insight and guidance that is transcendent of our physical circumstances. This is our transition point into the Symbolic mind.

The three stages of the dialogue follow this pattern:

Tribal: Your family may offer the position that "this illness is happening to all of us, and we will battle it together." Your physician may present data that reveals how other people have responded to treatment and coped. Through it all, the core position is that your illness is a group challenge, and the central question is "Why is this happening to us, and how are we going to handle it?"

Individual: The reality of what you are facing is seen as the individual challenge that it actually is: It isn't happening to "us," it's happening to "me." The question that surfaces next is often the most paralyzing: "What did I do to deserve this?" You feel that if you only knew why it was happening to you, you could cope with it. At this stage self-pity and depression can infiltrate your mind and become as great a crisis as the physical illness itself.

Symbolic: There remains one more position that can assist you more than any physical treatment: the capacity to respond Symbolically instead of literally to what is happening. Instead of asking "Why is this happening to me?" the deeper and more authentic questions to pursue are "*Why* is this happening? What is the meaning of this situation, and how can I best respond to it?" Conceive what is occurring to you to the most impersonal terms you can attain, and from that position, in that moment, consider what your most empowered responses should be. Think of your crisis as happening to someone you don't even know, and ask yourself how you would advise them. Refer to spiritual teachings that remind you that everything is for a reason and that having faith and trust in that reason makes the impossible quite possible.

From this position, you will be receptive to guidance and the clearest level of insight. From the Symbolic dimension, you can see your illness within the context of your whole life, far beyond what is happening in the moment. You become able to identify, understand, and dialogue with your archetypal patterns, seeing clearly those repetitive challenges that have formed the ongoing dynamics of your life. Through this process, you become better able to live comfortably with the mystery you have been dealt, because you now have a means by which to draw comfort from that mystery. The unanswered parts of your life no longer keep you stuck in your history, but become a rich lens through which you can know more about your own path of evolution. This is the climate in which genuine guidance thrives. The Symbolic mind carries the potential to reduce every fear within you to nothing more than meaningless words. With Symbolic sight, you can reenter the physical challenge of an illness armed with a sense of eternity.

Bearing in mind these three levels of power as a working model of your interior self, it's time to investigate your relationship to the mystery of healing.

◆

...AND HOW THEY CAN

Chapter Five

FINDING THE RIGHT PATH
THROUGH THE CHAOS
OF HEALING

Because our thoughts and emotions play a role in the development of an illness and because positive thoughts can increase our capacity to heal, the healing arts have turned from an exclusive focus on external medicines to a concern with one's internal, mental, and spiritual nature. Combining mind, body, and spirit in health practices has led to an embrace of diverse health treatments practiced in the East and West. The joined forces of complementary medicine and spirituality promise to be more effective in helping people heal terminal and chronic illnesses, maintain health well into the elder years, and retard the aging process. In addition, Eastern spirituality and the wisdom of native traditions from all cultures offer new views of a Divinity to Western cultures that had previously been influenced predominantly by the Judeo-Christian traditions. With so many choices suddenly floating into our field of vision, the challenge of healing can seem like an undifferentiated chaos. How do we wade through them to find the right healing path for ourselves? How do we find the right combination of inward spiritual practice and external treatments?

Begin by working to heal your spirit. A healthy spirit is essential for a healthy body, although a healthy spirit does not *guarantee* a healthy body. Understanding your spirit does hold the key to helping control what happens to your body and within it, however. Since many complementary medical treatments require you to be conscious of the role of the spirit in healing, you have to take personal steps to unite that belief and spirit with your body. In short, you need to physicalize your spirit, to embody it.

One way to do this is to practice your personal understanding of how your body and life reflect the energy of the chakras–sacraments–sefirot. This practice can help you give an energy form to your spirit and to your personal, inner Divine power. You will also need to release the outdated parent-child concept of an external God who operates on a reward-and-punishment system, the spiritual heritage of the Arien and Piscean ages. Recognize that a Divine force is intrinsic to your every thought and action, that an the inner force guides you to become ever more conscious. Getting to know better the nature of the God who is within reveals your own innate power and allows you to become aware of how you co-create whatever you experience in your life, including your health.

Fear interferes with the mindful use of your power. When you base choices on fears, chaos comes between you and your inner Divinity. To decrease your susceptibility to fear, your spiritual life requires attention and nurturing. You don't initially increase your spiritual power through business-as-usual, any more than you can enhance your culinary skills by playing the piano. The human spirit requires daily nurturing through a spiritual practice such as prayer or meditation. These practices nourish the energy system and help unite mind, heart, and spirit.

A spiritual practice is not the same thing, however, as living in a healthy way. Following either one path or the other does not accomplish both goals simultaneously. A healthy life includes getting enough exercise and the proper nutrition, avoiding toxic substances, and maintaining other conscious living habits. Healthy living, according to even the most stringent of rules, does not insure that an illness will not develop, however, but it certainly reduces the chances.

A healthy lifestyle helps you learn more about what your body requires for maximum physical well-being, and a spiritual practice furthers your understanding of the role the Divine plays in your life. It reveals the path you are meant to walk. Although a spiritual practice can help your spirit grow and improve your overall health by grounding and directing you to healthful, non-destructive behaviors, neither is it a guarantee of perfect health. As we have seen, it may even challenge you to endure an illness as the vehicle through which inspiration and a deeper sense of the power of your spirit can emerge.

When an illness is a part of your spiritual journey, no medical intervention can heal you until your spirit has begun to make the changes that the illness was designed to inspire. Medical intervention, complementary healing modalities, changes in nutrition, and overall lifestyle may all help to some extent and should certainly be used. But the most effective healing option, when you are facing an illness as a spiritual challenge, is to rely on your spiritual practice to bring you the insights you need. Your practice can be a means of enduring the disease and healing it through increasing the strength and wisdom of your spirit—or it can prepare you for the release of your life, if that is the Divine will for you. You need to redirect your faith from the physical realm to the spiritual realm.

Those who have been able to make this transition can become great inspirations to others. By examining how they have handled their crises, we may gain some insight into how to deal with our own.

Joseph Cardinal Bernardin, who for many years was the head of the Catholic Archdiocese of Chicago, is an example of someone who followed the path of illness in a conscious way. By doing so, he set an example for others that illness and even death are not to be feared. I'd like to look at the two years preceding his death from the perspective of the three forms of power discussed in the previous chapters. During those years, the Cardinal journeyed through all three kinds of power in an accelerated fashion.

In the early 1990s, a young man claimed publicly that he had been sexually exploited by Cardinal Bernardin. Although the Cardinal adamantly denied these charges, the accusations generated enormous scrutiny, suspicion, and criticism, especially given the number of sex scandals that had wracked the Roman Catholic priesthood in previous years. The Cardinal made every attempt to handle these charges with dignity. His public responses to his accuser were neither angry nor falsely compassionate. In the end, the young man recanted his charges, and the Cardinal made a public statement that he held no malice and forgave his accuser. He later met privately with the man.

Had Cardinal Bernardin functioned under Tribal power, he might have chosen to respond with legal action, a common Tribal response to an attack. From a Symbolic perspective, this was the Cardinal's "Judas" experience — a betrayal in public of all that his life's work stood for.

Soon after the resolution of the scandal, the Cardinal was diagnosed with pancreatic cancer. Although he worked to heal his illness, achieving a remission six months after his initial diagnosis, the illness returned. One could easily question why a man of such faith and spiritual support could not heal his illness, and suggest that his spirituality had failed him. But what if the Cardinal actually meant to die publicly, in order to show that dying can be an act of spirituality as much as living?

The Cardinal's illness could be Symbolically interpreted as his "crucifixion." All that the physical world could offer him, the best medical care, and the spiritual support of perhaps millions of people had failed. If he had remained attached to the physical world, he might have become a bitter man. But while he was dying from the cancer's recurrence, he chose instead to speak openly of his fear of death and his faith and, gradually, his acceptance of death. He authored a book entitled *The Gift of Peace*, to give hope and courage to people facing their own death or the death of a loved one. From a Symbolic perspective, his acceptance of his death is the ultimate act of forgiveness and the conscious release of his life to God. He showed others the way through the fearful corridor of death by courageously walking it himself, embodying an ultimate practice of spiritual healing. The message of hope that he left behind remains a real, living example of the spirit's power. We can even call it his "resurrection."

Seeing illness as a spiritual challenge does not reduce our chances of healing, but we need to understand that spirituality is first and foremost the path of gaining inner rather than physical strength. Physical healing can certainly follow, but whether it occurs or not is part of one's spiritual destiny.

I once knew an organic farmer named Jerry who could not comprehend the difference between spiritual practice and the need to respond to illness with a healing regimen. Jerry lived on a small farm so that he could grow his own food, and he was an expert vegetarian cook. He was also heavily into working out and had packed a room in his farmhouse with exercise equipment that he used two to three hours each day. Highly energetic by nature, he had a warm, sociable personality. Yet he was also angry. When he spoke to people about the necessity of learning the organic way of life, he would rave about the damage being done to the planet by people who had no awareness of the environment. His passionate approach to life carried a negative energy that made him despise the people who did not share his views.

At the age of 39, Jerry was diagnosed with bone cancer, a diagnosis that shocked him and everyone who knew him. His friends recommended every kind of healer they knew of, locally and nationally. He consulted with at least ten different healers, many of whom suggested a program that included getting more iron and amino acids into his system by eating some red meat. Jerry flatly refused. For him, eating meat would represent a violation of his lifestyle and his spirituality. The healers' recommendations infuriated him by implying that his choice of nutrition for so many years had been inadequate. Jerry's friends encouraged him to make the change in his diet, if only temporarily, to see if it could in fact make a difference. They kept telling him that he could always return to his vegetarian lifestyle once he was healthy again. But Jerry believed that his commitment to organic living was his spiritual expression and should be sufficient to get him back to health. He could not compromise on his dedication to being a voice for the environment, which he believed to be the sole path to consciousness.

As the months passed, Jerry's condition worsened. His friends begged him to seek out the assistance of people trained in spirituality to help him resolve the deep anger he was feeling. Jerry felt that God had betrayed him by giving him this illness, and that no spiritual director could explain why his healthy lifestyle had led to a terminal cancer when others who lived without any consciousness about their nutrition were thriving. The dilemma consumed his thoughts until it became an extremely negative obsession, displacing his attention to his own healing.

Jerry eventually passed away, believing until the day of his death that his life had been wasted, because all he had believed in, including the "God of the earth," had failed to heal him. Jerry's life, in contradistinction to Cardinal Bernardin's, reminds us to be careful not to confuse physical health with a genuine spiritual practice of compassion, prayer, and reflection. I am not saying that if Jerry had followed a prayer practice along with his meditative gardening and workouts, he would not have developed cancer or that he would have been able to heal his illness. A reflective, true spiritual practice, however, would have provided him with very different insights about his physical challenge. He might have been able to see that a variety of emotional and psychological choices were open to him.

Given Jerry's deep belief that organic gardening was itself a spiritual practice, he might have been able to bring a form of conscious meditation into his daily gardening routine, or he might have been inclined to spend more time in physical acts of prayer. He might have been able to recognize that anger is not the way to inspire people to realize the need to heal the earth. And he might even have come to see his challenge from a Symbolic perspective, in that he was experiencing the same toxicity as the earth he was working so hard to cleanse. This realization might have enabled Jerry to fight the illness more passionately, if only to become an even stronger environmental leader armed with deeper insights and inspiration.

Healing requires a willingness to make changes in both your physical and your spiritual ways of life. Healthy changes of lifestyle and spiritual practice are parallel roads leading to the same goal, and each road needs to be driven along every day. One of my workshop participants, Jeff, managed successfully to walk both of these roads. At the young age of 24, Jeff was diagnosed with a heart condition. At the time he was active in sports and bodybuilding and had just started a computer business. His diagnosis was that he essentially had a "hole" in his heart, which quite naturally shocked him and his family.

Before his diagnosis, Jeff had had no interest in spirituality. After discovering his condition, however, he learned everything he could about nutrition and the appropriate exercise practices for someone with his problem. Yet, as he put it, "I don't remember even having a spiritual word in my vocabulary at that time." One night, as he was drifting off to sleep, Jeff heard a voice that said, "Trust me." When he told me about this incident, he said that the voice was both loud and soft at the same time. He said that all he could think of was "Trust whom? Who is speaking to me?"

The next day, Jeff could not get his mind off the voice—or the next day, or the day after that. After thinking about the directive for a week, he passed by a church during his daily walk. "I didn't even pay attention to what denomination the church was," he recalled. "All I know is I walked in and sat in the front pew. I looked at the cross hanging on the wall and said out loud, 'Was that you talking to me?' And then, suddenly, I knew it was."

Jeff left that church filled with a deep belief that some Divine force was involved in what was happening to him. He began a daily ritual of prayer and started to seek out the company of those who "spoke spirituality." One of the most surprising things he encountered among the people he met was that when he shared the experience of hearing a nocturnal voice, no one questioned its authenticity. In fact, he said, they treated it as if it were the most normal thing in the world.

Jeff learned about meditation and visualization and found enormous comfort in many books on spiritual topics. Although he had never before considered that he needed to feed his spirit as well as his body, he became dedicated to doing both each day. He actually reached a point where he felt that whether he lived or died was no longer the challenge he was facing. Instead, what counted for him was how well he could face either option, without knowing what lay ahead for him.

Within two years, Jeff's heart condition was fully healed, much to the surprise of his physicians, who told him that recovery in such cases was rare. By that time, he had come to a place of deep inner contentment. "At work, people come to me to calm down," he said. "They tell me that talking to me seems to help them see things more clearly and not to feel so upset about small incidents that happen each day. I feel like a counselor or a therapist, which is fine, though I never expected to play that role. I believe that I am meant to help people in just this way, quietly giving them positive thoughts and hope that tomorrow will be a better day. Symbolically, I now believe that this is the reason my illness was a heart disorder. I think it opened my heart."

ILLNESS, PERSONAL INTIMACY, AND THE FEAR OF HEALING

True healing is one of the most frightening journeys anyone can undertake. For some people, illness can provide a feeling of physical safety that sometimes allows them to slow down the speed at which their lives are moving or changing. Illness can also offer the safety of not having to confront your inner issues or change yourself. And, as I have already noted, when you become seriously ill, you may experience a level of concern and attention from others that you might not otherwise receive. All this wonderful care and attention can be seductive and can subtly implant in you the belief that if you ever get well, you will lose it.

I have already pointed out that the study of archetypes, as they emerge in the examination of ourselves and our life patterns, can be the doorway into the biggest, brightest spaces of human consciousness. Yet I can now admit that I myself did not feel this way until illness compelled me to confront my own patterns and fears. Through that long, painful journey, I developed the intuitive ability to perceive these patterns in other people.

In 1982 I moved to New Hampshire to help start Stillpoint Publishing Company. As I mentioned in Chapter 1, the three of us who founded the company wanted to specialize in publishing books that furthered the human consciousness movement, but for me, that represented a professional goal rather than a personal commitment to a more conscious life. Prior to becoming involved in holistic health, I had worked as a journalist in Chicago and enjoyed perfect health—while living an unhealthy life. I smoked, drank coffee by the gallon, never exercised, and had absolutely no consciousness about what I ate. I didn't drink or take drugs, but given everything else I did, I certainly had enough toxins in my system without their help. Shortly after arriving in New Hampshire, I began to experience chronic lower back pain. It became so intense that sometimes I had to go to my chiropractor twice a day. I am still grateful to her for lowering her fee for me because I went so often—kind of a bulk discount.

I also developed endless headaches—migraines, sinus, and stress headaches. Some of them would last for a day, others for a week. I especially recall one headache that lasted for five weeks straight without letting up. I thought that was the worst one I would ever have, but I was wrong. A few years later, I actually had a headache that lasted continually from the month of May until the end of August.

During the onset of this headache pattern, I also developed chronic fatigue syndrome, which doesn't surprise me now, since the three of us were working virtually around the clock to get our company off the ground. As a result of the hours we kept and the continual pain I was in, my sleeping patterns became erratic. I would often spend half the night vomiting from pain, and then, in an extremely weakened condition, I would go into the office the next day and put in another ten or twelve hours, drinking endless cups of coffee to keep me going.

Around this time, the "wounded child" archetype became popular in books and in the psychological marketplace. I listened continually to people describing their inner child and blaming their behavioral patterns on the wounds their inner child had not yet processed. I thought they were all nuts, and given my penchant for blunt remarks, I frequently told them so—earning me the reputation of the person *not* to speak to in a crisis.

During the height of my chronic fatigue syndrome, a very close and dear friend of mine named Sally suggested that she take me to a healer she knew quite well. "And what is he going to do for me?" I asked in my tactful way. She said that he could heal people with his hands. I told her what I thought about that suggestion—again in blunt language—and we dropped the subject until a day came when I could not get out of bed. I phoned Sally that morning and asked her to make arrangements for me to meet with this healer. I added that she would have to pick me up since I was too weak to drive.

Within an hour of that phone call, we were off to meet with her healer. Sally spent the entire trip telling me of his ability and of her faith in him. When we arrived at the cabin he had set up as his office, he called me into the room where he saw his patients. He asked me what was wrong, and I told him that I was out of energy and that I simply needed to be "jump-started." He looked at my eyes, and then he looked over my head. After he made that same motion with his eyes about three times, he leaned back in his chair and folded his arms. "I refuse to help you," he announced. He then showed me to the door, commenting that I would be back to see him again. I told him to hold his breath until hell froze over, then left his office feeling totally abandoned by God and more alone than I can describe.

Sally was shocked when I told her what had happened. As we drove home, she kept apologizing for his behavior, and although I assured her that it wasn't her fault, I could see guilt written all over her face. We fell into several minutes of silence, and then Sally said in a soft voice, "I think you need to get in touch with your inner child."

That, of course, was about the worst thing she could have said to me, and definitely at the worst time. "I do not want to hear a word about that inner child nonsense!" I half screamed. "My inner child—if there is such a thing—is not wounded. I did *not* have a bad childhood, I do *not* come from a broken home, my parents still love each other deeply, and they have always loved my brothers and me. So exactly where would this inner child of mine have gotten any wounds?"

Sally suggested that wounds come in many forms during childhood and that regardless of how happy my childhood might have seemed, we all acquire some form of wound during our early years. I warned her that her head was getting filled with nonsense and suggested that she snap out of it.

After she dropped me off at my home, I went into my bedroom, fell on my bed, and sank deeply into the waste dump of self-pity. I felt that I had the right to feel sorry for myself, because here I was spending my life trying to heal others through publishing books on alternative health practices, but when I needed help most, the whole alternative world was failing me.

I remained in my black hole of self-pity until about ten days after my encounter with this healer. When Sally felt comfortable enough to ask him why he had refused to help me, he informed her that he had seen a presence standing behind me that had told him not to touch me. This bizarre revelation, when Sally repeated it to me, did little to clear up my funk. But a few days later, a group of students who were working with this man learned that in addition to his so-called healing practice, he had been molesting some of his female clients. When I heard that, I was awestruck by the notion that during the very time when I thought I had been abandoned, I had actually been protected. Yet in spite of this rather remarkable incident, I was still unable to heal, and my self-pity soon returned.

In 1985, as an emerging medical intuitive in the publishing business, I had begun to receive invitations in the New England area to lecture on the connection between energy and disease. Shortly thereafter, I was scheduled to give a workshop to a wonderful group of dentists in northern New Hampshire. My teaching style includes the use of case histories and anecdotes from people with whom I've worked, but because my experiences with others were minimal at that time in my career, I spoke about my own illnesses. One especially insightful dentist raised his hand after I had been talking about myself for a while. "How is it," he asked, "that someone your age gets so many childhood illnesses?"

I immediately felt as if this inner child, the one I thought I never had, had jumped out directly from my solar plexus, looked me square in the eye, and laughed in my face, as if to say, "And all this time, you thought it was *you* who ran your life! Well, toots, think again."

I was simultaneously stunned, upset, confused, and intrigued. After the workshop ended, I pondered this experience and its significance. As I slowly took a serious look at my inner child, I could perceive areas of my life that needed further exploration.

My headaches continued, however, until by the late 1980s, I believed that I would never be rid of them. All the while I was teaching more and more people in larger workshops all over the country, and my main theme was that it is possible to heal any illness. As I said those words out loud to a group, I would think to myself, "Except for me." I would often walk off a stage feeling like a fraud or, at the very least, like someone in a state of deep conflict. Although I genuinely believed in what I was teaching, I could not seem to connect with the power that underlay my words and ideas. I felt a little like the scholars in India known as *pandits*, who study and interpret the Hindu scriptures and all the subtleties of mystical practice but rarely seek the realizations they teach about. In short, I was unable to make healing work for me.

Then in August 1988 I had to undergo a relatively simple nose surgery. I returned to my hometown of Chicago for the operation, because I needed the rest. I knew that after the surgery, I would look like I had been mugged, and I felt it was wise to stay with my parents during my recovery. Two weeks after the surgery, which was successfully completed, I returned to my farmhouse in New Hampshire. No sooner had I walked in the front door than my nose started to bleed, slowly at first. I thought it odd, since I had never had a nosebleed before, even as a child.

The bleeding rapidly became a flood, pouring out of my nose and down my throat. I ran into my bathroom and vomited blood all over the walls and floor. I called my neighbors, Karol and Ray, who took me to their home, propped me up on their couch, and gave me an enormous bowl to catch the blood as it was flowing out of me. Karol said to me in her sweetest mothering tone of voice, "Now just relax, honey. No one ever dies from a bloody nose."

After the bleeding had continued for forty-five minutes, though, I heard Ray whisper to Karol, "We need to call for an ambulance." By the time the rescue squad arrived, I was too weak to move. They carried me into the ambulance, and two women were already in the back waiting to take care of me on our ride to the hospital. I had to sit up by this point because I was now choking on the blood that was flowing down my throat. As I did, I heard one of the women say to the other, "Do you think she's going to make it?"

At that remark, I looked out the window of the van, and then my head fell into the bowl of blood on my lap. Suddenly I felt myself floating outside the van, looking in at these two women, trying desperately to lift my head out of the bowl. I somehow knew that I was either dead or having a near-death experience. As I was floating away from the van, I moved farther and farther away from the earth until I was suspended in space. All of a sudden, I felt embraced by a loving and oddly familiar presence that told me that it wasn't yet time for me to come home, and that I needed to return because I still had work to do.

I was shown some images of what lay ahead for me, although they were vague and seemed almost like looking through air. As I was preparing to go back—assuming that I was actually *going* back—I could see my body, but by now it looked no bigger than a grain of sand. Floating out in space, I felt as if I were the size of infinity itself, and I asked the obvious question: "How will I get back in that body? I won't fit."

The image of a genie entering a bottle flashed through my consciousness, and in that instant I was magnetically drawn down into my body, all the while thinking, "Is that what the image of a genie in a bottle represents? Is it the spirit entering the body?"

After that experience, I took an even more serious look at my inner child. In the process, I realized that the reason I did not want to go inside was that I feared old feelings, as if looking into my own interior would be like unlocking a box that had been buried for thousands of years. Different images were arising in my consciousness. My dreams changed from fairly ordinary ones, rehashing everyday events, to images of a frightened child trying to walk confidently among a world of adults. I gradually realized that I had felt this way all of my adult life to that point. As I began to grasp the magnitude of my own sense of inadequacy, I was able to understand why I always seemed to play the "child" role in most of my working relationships. I knew nothing about what personal boundaries meant, and I often responded to challenging situations with sarcastic remarks—a juvenile method of communication that I had developed because I had not yet learned how to speak up for myself. I did see, however, that to heal my physical problems, I would first have to confront my inner child and heal the patterns of fear that this archetype represented in my own consciousness.

I did not want to do this inner work—first, because I knew it would not be easy, and second, because I was in for a long ride to the end of the line. At this writing I have not yet reached the end of this line, but I am many miles from the beginning. Through this experience I finally did connect with the energy of healing that had seemed so unattainable for so many years. More than simply believing in the existence of archetypal energies, I now know they are real. I know that they are not just abstract places we have invented to describe imaginary forces at work within us. These very real energies exist in every one of our thoughts and experiences.

Many of us fear, as I did, becoming intimate with our inner selves. Humbling and humiliating as it is, enlightening and terrifying as it may be, such intimacy is nevertheless an experience that happens to be essential to healing. If nothing else, healing requires personal honesty, and few things are more intimate.

THE TERMS OF BECOMING HEALTHY

Armed with the knowledge of my own resistance to the journey of healing, I decided to ask the participants of a subsequent workshop how important becoming healthy was to them. At first, everyone responded enthusiastically that nothing stood in the way of achieving this goal. But they answered so quickly and so ardently that I knew something was wrong; their response had been mental, not authentic and emotional. The emotional level reveals our true feelings.

I decided to test them by asking them to be specific about the possible changes in lifestyle that they would be willing to make in order to heal. Healing has its price, just as seeking to understand the nature of one's consciousness does. The price of becoming healthy is, in many respects, similar to the answer to another question I could have asked: "What are you willing to give up to meet God?" Abraham was asked to sacrifice his son. The requirement to give up something is symbolic of our agreement to release our allegiance to the dimension of physical authority; it is the test of our trust in the Divine. This test surfaces again and again as we meet every new challenge in our lives. We are not tested only once; we are continually confronted with the question "Which world is it that you trust, yours or Mine?"

With that in mind, I asked the group a series of questions, ratcheting up the level of commitment with each one.

"If healing required changing your job, would you do it?"

Most of the members replied yes.

"If healing required moving to another part of the country, would you do it?"

Again, most replied yes.

"If healing required that you change most of your attitudes toward others and yourself, would you do so?"

Now the group became more selective, pondering with a bit more thought. The responses varied more this time, with some people saying that they didn't think their attitudes needed that much changing. Others said that if such a level of change were needed, they would give it a try.

"If healing required you to change all of your physical habits, such as restricting what you could eat and adding an intense exercise program to your daily schedule, would you do that?"

Once again, people were selective in their answers. Some said that they would not want to give up certain things and couldn't see why they should. And when it came to the notion of a daily exercise program, several said that as much as they would like to add that discipline to their lives, they lacked the time.

"If healing required that you be alone for a long period of time, perhaps entering into an extended retreat, enabling you to confront the shadow side of yourself, would you do it?"

Now the answers got more interesting. Some members actually grew defensive: Why would I have to do something like that? they wanted to know. Others flat out said no, they would not do that—as if they feared that a positive response would automatically schedule them for a three-month retreat right after the workshop.

"If healing your emotional and psychological nature required that you experience a physical illness, perhaps a long and difficult one, as the means of contact with these parts of yourself, would you accept that challenge?"

The majority answered no. Some said they might if they had no other choice. Only one replied, "Absolutely."

"If the goal of becoming healthy required you to lose everything familiar to you—home, spouse, job, what then would you say?"

This time the group fell silent. No one wanted to answer. I knew they were frightened. When I asked them what they were afraid of, some of them responded slowly with questions that boiled down: "Why does healing an illness require so much loss and work? Why can't it be easy?"

My point in asking these questions, I told them, was neither to scare them nor to make the journey to health look like a bed of hot coals. It was to illustrate that we hold within us—whether or not we realize it—the terms upon which we will move forward with our lives, including the goal of healing an illness. Answering these questions, even while they were in a state of relatively good health, was clearly intimidating for them. Now, I suggested, imagine how you would feel if you really *had* to face this challenge. That much I could have answered for them.

A woman named Meg, for whom I had recently done a health consultation, was suffering from constant extreme pain in her middle back. She also felt a burning sensation in both her thighs that was so severe, she actually produced what appeared to be third-degree-burned flesh. Her feet had swollen to the point where she could no longer walk. By the time we spoke, her voice was weak, and it was apparent that she had been crying. As I did a reading on her, I sensed that she had just gone through a breakup with a man with whom she was deeply in love, someone she had counted on being her life partner. Symbolically, this represented someone she could "lean" on. In a rather confused way, Meg confirmed this, saying that yes, she had just parted with a man she had been dating for two years, and that yes, she had hoped it would work out in terms of a marriage—but not really.

I then asked her if she had felt sexually inadequate in the relationship, since an extreme sense of inadequacy seemed to be part of her dilemma. She said that she had never felt that way. I replied that some deep sense of inadequacy had to be a part of this situation, given the location of her back pain and the intense burning she was experiencing in her legs. She then said, "I didn't have enough money for him. He wanted a millionaire, and I can barely pay my own bills."

Despite his attitude and her illness, Meg was still seeing him. "He comes over every day to see how I'm doing," she said, "and I need him to do this, because I don't have anyone else where I am living who can help me."

I offered Meg a profile of the "terms" that her healing might require, headed up by moving away from this community in which she was without support from family or friends, or at the very least never seeing this man again. She remarked that neither was possible, especially never seeing him again.

I then asked her if she thought that becoming healthy meant that this man would no longer have a reason to visit her. Meg's response was so rapid that I don't think she realized what she said. "I can't get healthy. He would leave me and find someone else, and then what would I do?"

I asked Meg to try to look at her situation Symbolically, to imagine that her ex-boyfriend represented her fear of ending up alone in her later years, as she already was in her fifties. I suggested that by confronting this fear and learning that she could rely on herself, she would feel more confident and healthy. She might then also attract to herself a partner of equal strength. I asked her to imagine that she was living the myth of a "damsel in distress waiting for her knight in shining armor," who would come and take her to his safe castle. Then, instead of seeing her ex-boyfriend as a knight, she should see herself in that role.

She could not see herself or her ex-partner Symbolically in these ways. "He's not in my imagination," she said. "He's real. What possible good would it do for me to imagine him as Symbolic?"

Meg was so deeply embedded in Tribal consciousness that I could only communicate with her using Tribal language, so I suggested that she "temporarily" move in with a family member who could help nurse her back to health, even though her brothers and sisters lived in other states. She said she would give that some thought, comforted by the word *temporarily*.

Not everyone is so confined by their Tribal energy. A man named Tod wrote to me saying that after listening to me lecture on the terms we place on healing, he began to question seriously his own terms. Through this self-analysis, Tod realized that his prostate cancer had probably been created, in part, by his fear of his family finding out that he was gay. He had always kept this part of his life a secret and felt that if his family found out, they would be ashamed of him. He realized that his fear of their shame was also due in part to his own discomfort about his sexuality, and that unless he "came out of the closet," he would be interfering with his own healing.

So Tod had his family over for dinner, and after dinner he asked them if there were any conditions under which they would not love him. They were shocked by that question, and then his sister said, "You mean would we still love you if you told us you were gay?"

Tod was absolutely stunned by her response and the casual way she delivered it. "Yes," he said, "that's exactly what I mean!"

"And then," Tod wrote to me, "my sister said, 'Oh, we've always known that. It's no big deal. Is there anything else you wanted to tell us? I mean, are you robbing banks or something?' I started to laugh and cry at the same time. I felt the most enormous surge of love and gratitude toward my family. I can't begin to tell you how much I love my parents and that crazy sister of mine. And after that, I felt as though healing my body was also going to be, in my sister's words, 'no big deal.'"

We cannot heal serious or chronic illnesses without changing some part of our life pattern, and change is, without a doubt, the most frightening challenge in healing. Of course, not all changes are difficult, frightening, or painful. Many are actually quite pleasant, such as conducting your life at a less hectic pace and giving yourself more leisure time. Getting into a regular exercise routine and eating healthful food can also be enjoyable, once these activities become a natural part of your life. But these changes are all physical or Tribal.

Fear doesn't kick in until the level of change enters the Individual realm. Then we have to investigate what isn't working for us emotionally, psychologically, and spiritually. At this level we begin to generate a conditional, bargaining approach to healing.

When I asked my workshop participants what changes they would be willing to make for healing, the most telling response came from a woman I'll call Marta. "I'd like not to have to work full time," she said, "since I enjoy my free time too much. And I would like to have long vacations every year. I'd also like to be able to travel a lot, because that's one of my favorite things to do. And of course I wouldn't want my marriage to break up or to have to leave my children. I consider that completely unacceptable." Most of the things she named weren't aspects of her life she would sacrifice for healing, but wishes for things she didn't have at all.

After Marta finished, most of the group members jumped in with similar comments expressing an unwillingness to give up much at all for healing. Her bluntness had given them permission to withdraw from the positive responses they had tentatively given earlier. They were relieved to be able to avoid the possibility of facing tough choices.

Unfortunately, you cannot place your own terms and conditions on healing. Finding the right healing path requires all or nothing. Once you place conditions on healing, all you can achieve is conditional healing.

DEPENDENCE AND THE ASSUMPTION
THAT SOMEONE ELSE CAN DO IT FOR YOU

We are, by nature, dependent creatures—which isn't all bad. It's comforting to know that we can rely upon others and that they can count on us. We learn this as Tribal beings, gathering around weaker members to protect them. Healing, however, is one of the life challenges—perhaps the most extreme challenge—into which we must ultimately enter alone. Others can certainly offer their support, but only the ill person can accomplish the hardest and deepest work.

The positive attitudes that people hold for you during your healing simply are not sufficiently strong to improve your body physically, especially if you are being swamped by the fears an illness can generate or are taking a passive approach. One woman I met through a workshop was suffering from lupus and severe depression. I spoke to her about the need to retrieve some level of hope. "I leave the hope part up to my friends and my church," she said. "I have enough to do just getting up in the morning."

This is a classic example of a person relying on the Tribal will to do her own inner work. For all the comfort friends and family can bring, that power is diminished when the recipient does not try to help herself.

In another situation, I suggested to a man who was coping with prostate cancer and depression that he allow himself one hour a day of "depression" time. During this hour, I said, he should allow himself to cry, or scream, or beat up a mattress—anything to release the rage, fear, and grief that contribute to the force of depression. But after that hour, he should enter into prayer, meditation, or inspirational reading to get himself back to a place of hope. In this way, when he gathered with his friends or family members for their loving and positive support, he would be far more able to absorb the strong energy that they were transferring to his system.

As much as we would like others to be able to "take up our beds and walk" for us, they cannot. We can always be open to others' love and support, but the actual work that needs to be done can only come from within ourselves.

COMPLEMENTARY TREATMENTS

Being diagnosed with an illness can quite understandably produce massive confusion. Like waking up in a strange country to which you don't remember traveling, you may well feel that you do not know what to do or to whom to turn for help. A closed mind is not an asset. Be open to any and every option that can help you. Since the emergence of the holistic approach to healing, it has become popular in alternative healing circles to take a negative view of allopathic medicine. In fact, many people who are engaged in an alternative healing program express hostility toward any support from conventional medicine. In the long run, this can be a mistake. Strong negative feelings about or fears of allopathic medicine are not a good reason to rule them out. Your healing efforts can end up as attempts to run away from conventional medicine more than as attempts to run toward the improvement of your health. If you decide to go holistic, you need to do so after serious research into the full spectrum of the options available in both medical arenas. But keep in mind that in many cases, the most effective course of action is to combine the best of both worlds.

In any event, the image of allopathic medicine as the enemy is no longer valid or useful. Although the medical establishment initially resisted alternative healing modalities, it has made a major shift in recent years in opening itself to reflexology, chiropractic, massage, and acupuncture; the use of vitamins, enzymes, amino acids, and other vital supplements; and the use of nutritional treatments to combat free radicals, the elements in the body that support the development of illness. Fortunately, allopathic and complementary medicine have begun to join forces in a way that mirrors the merger of opposites characteristic of the

Aquarian age. The advantage to remaining open to both medical possibilities is a much wider range of healing energy from which to choose.

Speaking of choices, the wisest decision you can make after receiving an initial diagnosis is to get a second and even a third professional opinion. Bear in mind that each physician has a different history of treating each illness, and so the chances are that each one will have somewhat different suggestions. Although this variety may initially seem to complicate your decision making, it is more helpful in the long run because having a variety of options represents hope. In my own case, when I was seeking help for debilitating headaches including migraines, I met with one physician who was an "expert" in the treatment of sinus conditions. After examining me, he said — and this is a direct quote — "I can do nothing for you. You have nothing to look forward to but a life of relentless pain." Had I listened to him, I would have been devastated, not to mention that his words would have contributed to implanting an extremely negative thought in my consciousness.

Instead, I decided to check out other professional resources, both allopathic and holistic, then combined the best of both for my treatment program. Ultimately, by following the advice of a wonderful physician and a gifted chiropractor, I found a way out of a condition that had caused me years of pain. But I had to look beyond the prognosis of the original physician. That experience taught me how susceptible we are to the opinions of the so-called experts; an opinion is merely one person's perception and should never be taken as the "last word" in any situation.

When faced with a diagnosis of a breast or ovarian tumor, many women take the position of not wanting to be "cut up" through surgery. Cindy, a woman I met a few years ago, decided to treat her malignant breast tumor with every alternative medical treatment available. Her malignancy was particularly brutal in that it penetrated her skin, causing constant bleeding and excruciating pain. When none of her options led to any improvement, she went to see a physician who specialized in low-grade chemotherapy combined with various energetic treatments. Her tumor was reduced by fifty percent. Within two months, however, it had returned, and other growths had begun to show up as well.

Cindy then returned to the physician who had helped reduce her tumor, and though he put her under treatment again, he also suggested that she have these growths surgically removed. She refused even to consider that option. She believed that she had a strong enough mind and spirit to beat the illness, and she was repulsed by the thought of putting large amounts of chemicals into her body. When I had the opportunity to work with her, I received a very strong impression that most of her energy was not really in her body but was still in her marriage, which was rapidly declining. She said that her husband and his family had been highly critical of her growing interest in self-development. The atmosphere at home had become so unbearable, in fact, that she had finally moved out. Her efforts to meet with her husband during the following year, in hopes of a reconciliation, were rejected. She was left with the impression that he had really wanted her to move out for a long time but had lacked the courage to say so directly, and so he had forced her to make the decision by making her life with him uncomfortable. Because she was the one to move out, it appeared that it was she who wanted the divorce.

I explained to Cindy that she was directing the energy she required to heal herself toward healing her marriage instead. Her body was unresponsive to all of her efforts to heal because what little energy remained there was not strong enough to work with the natural treatments. It would be far more helpful to her, I said, if she would work with a counselor who could help her release the anger she was holding inside toward her husband and his tribe and move forward with her own life. Since her rage and her marital situation were totally consuming her life-force, she needed to reconsider allopathic treatments. This would be difficult for her, however, since it would seem to be admitting to her husband and his "tribe" that they had been right all along about her "crazy" interest in personal development. Nonetheless, she had to do it.

To make a transition in our lives, we need to release something from our past—a symbolic lightening of our energy. In Cindy's case, the release of her past meant leaving a tribe that could not support the person she wanted to become. When I explained this to her, Symbolically it made sense to her, but she could not actually make emotional contact with the image. While her mind found great comfort in the idea of entering into Individual power, her energy was unable to make the transition. Eventually her cancer spread throughout her body, and she passed away within a year of her original diagnosis.

In a workshop I gave two years ago, a woman named Mary Ellen told of her healing process. After she had been diagnosed with thyroid cancer, her physician recommended that she undergo radiation therapy. She said that she would give it some thought. "At first, everything he said terrified me," she told my workshop. "I couldn't picture myself going through radiation. I always thought of it as burning the skin off one's body. I was very familiar with alternative treatments, but not specifically for thyroid cancer. So I went to several holistic practitioners for advice and asked them what their success had been in treating other patients who had my condition. They shared their success stories along with reports on their patients whose cancer had spread, and the numbers seemed to be about equal. I guess I was disappointed, because I had expected to hear that everyone they treated had been cured, which, I admit now, was totally unrealistic on my part.

"The more I considered my situation, the more I thought that perhaps the best thing for me to do was to take the advice of both areas of medicine and combine them, which is exactly what I did. I took the radiation treatments, and I did acupuncture, therapy, nutritional changes, yoga—everything I could think of. Within six months, I got the report from my physician that my cancer was in remission. I told him that I preferred the word *healed*, and he said, 'I guess I would too.'"

Ultimately, the wisest path is to keep an open mind to any positive method of healing, regardless of whether it is allopathic or holistic. Any treatment that can enhance your healing and bring hope and strength back to your body is worth considering.

You can use visualization as a means of drawing together all the elements in your healing regimen. The most effective visualization I have ever worked with in this context begins by imaging yourself in the center of a wheel with many spokes. Visualize each of the spokes as representing one of the healing options you have chosen. For example, let one spoke be "prayer," another "talk therapy," another "acupuncture," "support group," "Therapeutic Touch," "skilled physician," and so on. You may visualize the actual words on each spoke, or some image representing that particular healing modality.

Now see yourself lying down or sitting in the middle of this wheel. Let the wheel begin to spin slowly around you. Visualize the energy from all of these healing techniques flowing into your system together—not as separate disciplines but as one enormous, integrated structure that is collectively radiating its power into your system. You may find that playing music is helpful in conjuring the movement of this wheel. Let yourself drift into the force of the wind that is generated by the spinning motion, a wind that is melting your physical body into fluid, draining from your system every toxin and every element of illness. Visualizing a spinning wheel is remarkably effective because it can actually generate heat in your body, creating a tangible manifestation of healing energy.

AVOID THE TEMPTATION
TO SPEAK WOUNDOLOGY

Before moving on to the methodologies for helping yourself heal, I'd like to bring your attention back to the subject with which I began: the dangers inherent in speaking woundology. Few situations in life can make you feel more utterly alone than the nocturnal dread that rises within you as the sun sets every evening on your unhealed body and soul. In response, making a strong connection to either the "martyr" or "victim" archetype can become hypnotic, while the temptation to become addicted to your support is equally powerful.

I was introduced to a woman named Belle through her husband, who contacted me because he was at his wit's end. Belle had broken her leg three months earlier. By now, he said, she should be back on her feet. Prior to her breaking her leg, however, Belle had announced to her family that she would no longer play the role of the family caretaker. She would no longer do the cooking and cleaning or any of the other household chores for her husband and their four children—two teenagers and two younger ones. After she broke her leg, her daily routine was to get dressed in the morning, sit in the same chair in her living room, and read or watch television. She laughed about her situation, telling her family, "See, even God wants me to just take it easy now. He agrees with my decision, and my broken leg is my proof."

Belle's husband tried to reason with her, but it was useless. He promised to take her on a wonderful vacation—which, for him, would be a substantial stretch of his financial resources—but even that did not move her, either literally or figuratively, from her position in that chair.

Then he told the children to stop cleaning and cooking to see if that motivated her. All that happened was that the house fell apart, and eventually he got fed up with taking the kids out for fast-food dinners. Nothing worked. He said he even considered moving out with the children, but he discarded that option since he couldn't really afford to support two households.

I offered this man a Symbolic perspective of his wife. I didn't actually think it would do much good, but I didn't know what else to say—if nothing else, I thought, it might add a bit of humor to a very dismal situation. I told him to think of her as a lazy queen. The family should stop directing all of their attention to her, I said, and instead focus on themselves and having fun together, leaving the "queen" to sit alone on her throne. Perhaps being left out of their playful activities would motivate her to want to be a part of the family again, since responsibility clearly held little appeal. He laughed for a moment at the thought of her being a lazy queen, saying that it suited her perfectly. But he doubted that family fun would be more appealing to her than her books and television, he said.

"Then take the television out of the house," I said. "In other words, limit the size of her 'court,' and that might limit her pleasure. If playful options don't motivate her, perhaps boredom will be more effective."

That was the end of our conversation. After thinking a moment, he said he would put the television in the basement. That way the kids could still use it, and if Belle wanted to watch it, she would at least have to walk down the stairs.

I believe this must have worked, since the man did not contact me again, but the outcome of the story is less important than the way it illustrates dramatically the power of woundology to control others.

In another workshop a man named Julio spoke up about his struggle with depression, and he recounted how his wife's determination to help him get out of it had finally worked. Julio would go in and out of depression on a regular basis, though it was particularly bad during the winter months. When he was in a depressed state, he would spend his weekends mostly in bed, getting up only for meals, and then he would sit in front of the television with a blank stare as he ate. His wife tried everything to help him cope with his condition. She would suggest that they go out for dinner or to a movie, or go away for the weekend just to get out, but he always shot down her suggestions.

"Finally," Julio said, "she hit the ceiling. She told me that I had become a self-centered bore and that she no longer cared how depressed I was. She was going to live a full life, with or without me. She started to go out with friends, not only on weekends, but often during the week as well. Half the time, I had no idea where she was.

"When she came home, she would tell me what a great time she'd had and then ask if I had enjoyed my evening with the television. Next she moved out of our bedroom, telling me that I no longer had the energy to arouse her. In fact, she said that I had become a twenty-four-hour bore. I told her I needed more time to heal, to which she replied, 'And I need the time to avoid getting ill, which means I have to avoid you. So take as much time as you need, because I've filled in those empty places that I used to share with you, and you know what? With each passing day, I miss you less and less, because you aren't a person anyone can miss very much.'

"I was hurt at first by her remarks, and then I got scared. I couldn't stand the thought of losing her, so I just made the decision to snap out of it, even if I had to fake the appearance of being out of my depression. I started to force myself to go out with her and do things together. It was very, very difficult at first, because I was still so depressed. It felt artificial to act as though I weren't depressed, but I didn't have any choice. In the long run, though, my determination actually healed my condition, because I began to feel that I was in charge of my moods instead of my depression controlling me. Now when I feel a mood swing coming on, I also feel that I have a choice to fight back. And I have my wife to thank for it."

When people allow a "victim" to control them because of an injury or an illness, or when "victims" align their personal suffering with an outside cause, they are reinforcing negative Tribal power. This power encompasses not only the victims but most of the people who may believe they are helping but are actually supporting the victim's negativity—or, in the language of twelve-step programs, "enabling" them.

I had the opportunity a few years ago to meet with a man who said he was suffering from Gulf War syndrome. Tyrone's body was weakening with each passing month. He had suffered a severe loss of hair and had chronic pain throughout his body, mostly in his legs, which made walking very difficult. He said that his condition had started about six months after he returned from the war.

"The army did this to me," Tyrone said, "and those bastards won't admit it. Not only should I receive financial compensation from them because I can't work anymore, I should also receive a public apology for what they did to me and to all the other guys in this situation. There are a lot of us, you know. I'm not the only one. And get this—when I went to the veterans hospital for treatment and told the doctors that I and a lot of other guys who were in that war had Gulf War syndrome, they told me that the disease did not exist. Do you know what that means? It means I'm imagining this whole thing. So I said to them, 'Well, if it isn't Gulf War syndrome, then what the hell is it?' They said that they weren't sure, but they suggested I take a lot of vitamins, eat better, and see a therapist. In other words, they were telling me that I was crazy."

I told Tyrone that I didn't think the insult was the issue so much as his anger and the fact that his condition had become a statement of his feeling of betrayal by the military—the Tribal power with which he most identified. He admitted that he did feel completely betrayed and abandoned by the army, and he said that he now felt he had an obligation to make them publicly admit that they had used chemical weapons that caused their own soldiers to become diseased. He was collecting the names and addresses of all the other men and women who had the same illness. He wanted them to join forces with him to get the media support that would, in turn, put pressure on the military to admit the truth. He had the full support of his wife, he said, who was doing all she could to assist him in bringing the reality of Gulf War syndrome to the public.

I asked Tyrone which goal was stronger, the desire to heal himself or the need to prove that the army had violated its own people. He replied that they were both his goals, and he wondered why he couldn't succeed at both.

I told him that succeeding at both would require that he change his state of mind from waging his "Tribal war" to doing all that he could to heal himself first. He would find far more support among those who had the same illness, I said, by becoming a person who had succeeded in healing the condition from which they all suffered. Then they would all want to know how he had managed to achieve his recovery.

Tyrone said that although that option made sense to him, if he did heal, he would no longer have any physical proof that he had ever had the illness, and therefore no one would believe him—least of all the military.

I pointed out that if he was determined to heal at the same speed as his "wounded Tribal comrades," he was, in effect, calibrating the speed and success level of his recovery to that of his entire Tribe. The choice to recover at the pace of a group is always risky, because it's such a mentally and energetically heavy path to walk. And if he did not recover, what good would his effort be in the long run?

I knew that what I had said to Tyrone clicked with his mind, but I could also see that his heart remained dedicated to his wounded Tribal comrades. I had no doubt that he would continue to try to prove the reality of his illness to military officials rather than direct his energy to healing his body. Since he was prepared to die for his cause, typical of the "martyr" archetype, shifting gears would be, for him, a betrayal of his wounded Tribe.

Let me emphasize again that the support of a group is essential to one's healing journey, but it has to be the kind of support that encourages movement in a positive direction. Realistically, allow yourself a few hours or one day a week to clear out your sad, overwhelming, and often depressing emotions about your illness, but after that embrace, once again, the energy of hope. This is where the loving support of friends and family members, along with professional intervention, becomes most effective—as a system through which the journey can become less onerous, helping your way back up to the light.

Keeping that in mind, let's explore the many options we do have that can help us along the path to healing.

Chapter Six

◆

IGNITING THE HEALING
FIRE WITHIN

It's one thing to understand intellectually the steps you need to take to heal. It's quite another to understand what you need to do on an emotional level. To ignite the healing fire, you need to believe something with your heart. The heart holds the catalyst that causes the rest of the bodymind to heal in a chain reaction.

The greatest illusion of the New Age is that awareness alone heals. Believe me, awareness by itself does nothing. The Hindus and Buddhists called what we see and perceive around us *maya*—illlusion. Relying on intellectual awareness alone to heal your body is wishful thinking. It is as delusionary as using cocaine, and more addictive; it makes you think that your life is changing even as it renders you more powerless. You don't need a wishbone; you need a backbone.

To begin to combine the power of mind, body, and spirit into a will to heal, let's learn how to use the three kinds of perceptions outlined earlier, and below, to change your mind—and change your life. Interpreting your thoughts, attitudes, and challenges within this three-part model of Tribal, Individual, and Symbolic sight will give you a powerful advantage for healing both physical problems and life crises. These ways of looking at life can give you three different perspectives on your healing

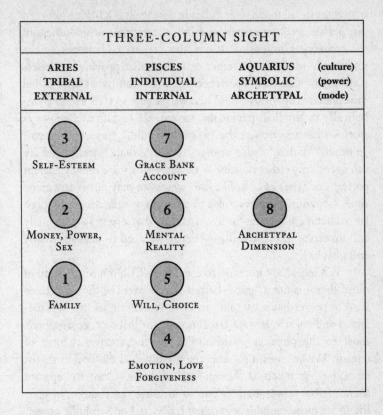

THREE-COLUMN SIGHT			
ARIES **TRIBAL** **EXTERNAL**	**PISCES** **INDIVIDUAL** **INTERNAL**	**AQUARIUS** **SYMBOLIC** **ARCHETYPAL**	(culture) (power) (mode)

3
 SELF-ESTEEM

7
 GRACE BANK ACCOUNT

2
 MONEY, POWER, SEX

6
 MENTAL REALITY

8
 ARCHETYPAL DIMENSION

1
 FAMILY

5
 WILL, CHOICE

4
 EMOTION, LOVE FORGIVENESS

challenge and a better grasp of what is happening to you and within you. As Carl Jung was fond of saying, no problem is resolved on the level at which it occurred; we must rise to a higher level to find a solution.

The three columns in the model represent the three forms of power (Tribal, Individual, and Symbolic) and the three astrological ages under which they developed. In each column are the chakras that correspond to each kind of power, and the area of life that relates to each chakra. These chakras are fairly self-explanatory, except for seven and eight. The "grace" or "cellular bank account" is where you store the energy, or grace, that you need to power and heal your body. I will discuss the eighth chakra in greater detail in Chapter 7, but in essence it is a bridge between our personal consciousness and the impersonal consciousness of the archetypal dimension. It contains archetypal patterns, or the universally recognized themes or images that provide an impersonal view of human experiences, derived from what Jung called the collective unconscious. When we are able to view events Symbolically rather than personally, we can see certain archetypes at work within us, such as the "wounded child," "rescuer," "hero," "mother," "father," "wise woman," or "wild man." Archetypes are not necessarily either positive or negative—they are merely ancient patterns or types of behavior into which we may fall at any given time. Looking at our response to an event as reflecting a particular archetype allows us to avoid taking that event so personally and investing in it the cellular energy we need to heal spiritually and physically.

While you are learning to use Three-Column Sight, keep in mind that it is not a "good–better–best" system of thought. Each kind of power has something to offer in helping us live in a balanced and conscious way. Tribal power, for instance, corresponds most to the physical world and is the most external form of energy. We are meant to embrace the physical dimension that it embodies, as much as the spiritual dimension, not to separate them. Tribal power enables you to measure the changes in your life in far more tangible ways than Individual or Symbolic power. But tribal power can also limit your ability to heal if you allow yourself to think conditionally (for example, "If this drug works, then maybe this illness can be healed"). For that reason, you have to manage this level of consciousness carefully. You might practice thinking, "This healing treatment will work for me because I know what my body needs." Keep tabs on each time you have a negative Tribal thought, such as "I'm not sure this will do any good," and when you find yourself with such a thought, consciously call on your fifth chakra energy ("will" or "choice") to say, "I make the choices I need," and feel confident that those choices will work for you. If you find yourself thinking or believing that illness heals only through drugs, you need to call on your Individual willpower to decide, for instance, "Anything can be healed, and I can achieve the most complete healing."

Using Individual and Symbolic power frees you of the pre-conceptions and temporal limitations of your external environment. Symbolic power allows you to see through physical illusions and recognize the lesson being offered by each challenge you face. By ascending to a Symbolic level, where time and space are not subject to human limitations, you can see things from this higher perspective. You are then in a position to chart a course of action, using Individual willpower. You can use the energy of Symbolic sight in all aspects of your life, from creating a new job to letting go of the past and moving on.

The first step in using Three-Column Sight is to empty yourself of negative belief patterns about healing. Start by making a chart with room for three columns, and write the names of the three kinds of power at the top of the columns. Identify two or three of your core beliefs that are related to Tribal and Individual perception and power, and write them down in the appropriate column in the chart. These beliefs may be either negative or positive. For example, "Healing is painful, long, and difficult" is a negative belief pattern that flows from Tribal power, and so you should list it in the Tribal column. The belief "Illness holds a message of change for me, and I need to be receptive to whatever change is necessary" is an outgrowth of Symbolic power, because it creates a state of mind that is receptive to detachment, to seeing things in archetypal rather than personal terms. So it should be listed in the Symbolic column.

Here are ten examples of beliefs for each kind of power. The reason the Tribal beliefs are all negative is that Tribal culture is more inclined to hold on to negative beliefs than are the other two, although Individual power also holds on to a few somewhat negative beliefs. As you mature in spiritual sight, you will be better able to realize the inherent power within yourself (Individual) as opposed to seeking power outside yourself (Tribal).

Tribal Beliefs About Healing

1. Illness is a long and painful process.
2. Serious illness cannot be fully healed.
3. Only chemical medicine is effective.
4. Illness is the result of stress directed toward me from other people.
5. I had nothing to do with the creation of this illness.
6. I am being punished for something I did wrong.
7. Turning to therapy means admitting to having a mental illness.
8. My doctor is responsible for my healing.
9. Illness has nothing to do with my emotions or psychological state.
10. Bargaining with the Divine is necessary for my healing.

Individual Beliefs About Healing

THE NEGATIVE SIDE OF THE INDIVIDUAL MIND

1. My illness is the result of negativity.
2. My illness must involve a karmic factor.
3. Allopathic medicine negates the power and effectiveness of holistic medicine.
4. Meditation and nutrition offer enough support to heal my illness.
5. My illness must be rooted in my childhood because my childhood was so painful.
6. I will be alone if I become a healthy and strong individual.

THE POSITIVE SIDE OF THE INDIVIDUAL MIND

7. Healing is a spiritual journey.
8. My spirit is stronger than my physical body.

9. There are lessons I must learn as I work through the process of healing.

10. Healing requires that I take responsibility for the process.

SYMBOLIC BELIEFS ABOUT HEALING

1. I am a part of a universal system of life.

2. All that is life supports my life.

3. Identifying my archetypal patterns helps me to recognize my role in universally shared patterns.

4. Striving for the Symbolic meaning in the experience of an illness gives genuine support to the physical path I need to follow for my healing.

5. My illness may be a way of receiving a new spiritual direction.

6. Seeking negative reasons for why an illness has come into my life is ultimately of little value. All that truly matters are the choices I make today.

7. There are no wrong choices. Every choice I believe in is an effective means of healing.

8. I constantly receive guidance toward the meaning and purpose of life.

9. Time is an illusion and therefore has no power in the healing process.

10. Age holds no power in the healing process.

Now let's apply Three-Column Sight to a typical Tribal belief and see how we can transform it into a Symbolic perception. Begin by writing down the belief "Illness is a long and painful process" in your Tribal column. Then take it to the Symbolic level of perception, where time is not a factor and pain can be a teacher. Symbolic perception can dissolve the power of that Tribal belief by seeing it differently, so in your Symbolic column write, "Healing transcends linear time. It can occur in an instant." Now you need to build a bridge of action to connect those two polarities. In your Individual column, create the bridge by writing, "I commit to focusing my attention and will on maintaining my energy in the invisible moment of here and now." This means that every time you feel yourself slipping into a negative thought like "Why did this happen?" or listening to someone else voicing such a belief, you return to an inner mantra that reorients you immediately to the transcendent thought that the belief may be true for that person but not for you. This mantra could be as simple as saying, "That Tribal thought has no authority over me. I will not attach one of my circuits to that thought. I will not dissipate my energy in such thoughts."

As you seek to transform negative Tribal and Individual beliefs about healing into Symbolic ones, maintaining objectivity or detachment is the key. "My experience of illness" becomes "the experience of illness." At the physical level, learning something through illness is obviously a much more arduous process than learning it through reading a book. Yet on the Symbolic level, they both become simply experiences through which you learn. You have to get accustomed to viewing your own illness the way you would view yourself going back to school. In fact, reaching a detached state of mind for even five minutes a day is so valuable that it can infuse your body with the equivalent energy of six months of living in genuine hope.

Detachment is not easy to achieve. In Western culture the term itself can be negative, representing a cold and distant attitude, sometimes even involving distaste or resentment. In healing, it is wiser to think of detachment as a way of separating oneself from the fears of the mind and viewing your circumstance as an experience through which you are passing rather than as one that controls your physical life. One effective method of achieving this spiritual position is to create a mantra, prayer, or chant that helps you focus immediately on a transcendent perspective. For example, close your eyes and repeat a phrase such as "I am ascending beyond my fears in this moment and always" or "Fears no longer have authority over my spirit." You may turn to a spiritual figure who represents the state of consciousness you are seeking in that moment—whether it's Jesus, the Buddha, Mary, Ramana Maharshi, or Teresa of Ávila. The mantra or prayer need not be long and involved. In fact, the shorter the better; brevity holds power because short prayers are easier to repeat.

As you list your positive and negative beliefs in the columns most appropriate for them, try to estimate the degree to which you are energetically connected to each negative belief. Conversely, gauge the amount of energy you would like to transmit into each positive belief. The negative belief "Healing is painful, long, and difficult," for example, may hold a substantial amount of authority within you, whereas the more positive belief "I am capable of healing anything" may be something you would like to believe but are not yet able to own completely. In that case, make a notation that you would like to direct a major percentage of your energy into that belief pattern. You might also distinguish your connection to each belief just by writing "active" or "inactive" next to it. Try hard to distinguish when a belief is merely an intellectual idea to you and when it actually holds authority within you. As I said, intellectual ideas have no healing power whatsoever.

This exercise cannot be completed in one day or even in one week. Don't become frustrated if at first you can list only a few beliefs. It will take a great deal of conscious effort to unearth all the belief patterns to which you hold. Thoughts and attitudes will arise with the various situations and conversations of your everyday life, showing you your beliefs. Different people bring out different sides of you; some add fire to the hopeful side of your personality, while others activate your fears. Every belief pattern is worth examining, so keep a notebook with you at all times specifically for recording thoughts and memories that are triggered by this process. Keep in mind that negative beliefs usually result in negative behavior patterns. Work backward from the behavior patterns that trouble you until you discern the beliefs underlying them. For example, if you find that a recurring illness results from or is exacerbated by a diet loaded with refined foods and sugar, you may be able to trace this negative behavior—eating that diet—to the belief that you have nothing to do with the creation of your illness.

If you seem to hit a wall in coming up with your beliefs, try talking to a sibling or other family member about attitudes that you share and the differences between you. Keep the conversation neutral—you just want to learn more about your tribe's conscious and unconscious beliefs. Also, if you work in an office, ask your trusted co-workers or friendly professional colleagues about the kinds of beliefs that they think bind you and govern you at work. Although turning to other people for a "perception check" may seem an awkward task at first glance, you will find it useful in organizing your thinking about the issues that naturally arise in the healing process. For example, you may be in a working situation in which you feel that you haven't contributed as much to a project as your co-workers have. Is this an accurate assessment, or are you telling yourself this because you have always looked at yourself through the lens of inadequacy? Ask co-workers you can trust whether they feel the same way about themselves—or about you. If you believe that everything that has gone wrong on the job has always been your fault, ask if that is how they see you or if you are making a self-punishing assumption.

If you have a spiritual teacher or belong to a religious institution, seek out your priest, minister, rabbi, lama, or spiritual director and ask for help in exploring troubling questions such as "Have I failed to establish a connection with the Divine because I've never had a continual or classic spiritual practice?" An even more useful question might be "Can kindness toward others be considered a spiritual practice?" These questions, and the dialogues that result from reaching out to people for their opinions, can provide you with enormous comfort or guidance in creating a more positive direction for yourself.

The next step in Three-Column Sight is to examine your relationships with others. The purpose of this step is to help you evaluate how much energy you are still investing in your history, permitting it to drain away from your present life and health. Just as you estimated the amount of power you allot to your beliefs, you will now gauge the energy you are "giving away" to your relationships. Once you are conscious of damaging old connections, you can learn to stop making such bad energy investments. Remember that healing is an "energetically expensive" task, and you'll need to regroup all of your vital energy into your immediate, present "grace bank account." You have to be present to win—to heal.

List the relationships in your life that you feel are in some way incomplete, including the name of the person and the reason why. List past relationships, too, whether parental or sibling, friendly or professional, as they come to mind. You might list your mother or father, for instance, if you still feel that they have never accepted you for the person you have become. Perhaps one of your parents died when you were a child, leaving you with a sense of abandonment that has not yet healed. Or you may feel that you harmed one or both of your parents in some way, and you still retain a deep feeling of guilt. If you feel that your unfinished business with a parent commands a high percentage of your energy, then note that fact. You might use a phrase such as "major energy drain" or "minor energy drain" to distinguish among relationships.

You need to bring the same kind of attention to all the other relationships that still contribute a negative influence to your life—business associates, romantic connections, friendships that have failed. Note how much negative energy you are generating toward people you envy or fear. With each one of these relationships, make certain that you also identify the type of negative feeling you associate with them—the reason you are still transmitting your energy in their direction. Finally, if you have any negative associations with physical places, whether cities or countries or even the schools you have attended or the houses and neighborhoods in which you once lived, follow the same process of energy evaluation.

As a rule, most of your negative associations will fall into the Tribal column. Much of the pain we receive and generate comes from problems in our childhood years, our relationships, and our occupation. We have issues around money, power, sexuality, and self-esteem. Although the journey of life is essentially spiritual, we discover our spirit through experiences in the physical world. The stronger and more conscious you become in your spirit, the more you can return that positive energy to the material realm, the world around you, your relationships, family, and profession.

Finally, you can apply Three-Column Sight to your behavior patterns, using the same method. One form of Symbolic reasoning is to identify archetypal patterns active within you, such as your "wounded child" or "rescuer." Using an archetypal approach allows you to recognize your own behavior from a more detached and compassionate position. List some of your own issues regarding money, sex, and power. Do you have trouble holding on to money? Or do you use sex as a way of avoiding intimacy? Are you afraid to exercise power because your father was overbearing, or do you use it inappropriately for the same reason? Note again that most of these behavior issues fall into the Tribal column, even issues such as being unable to forgive someone. Suppose you have this problem: Although forgiveness is a matter of the heart (fourth chakra), the reason you cannot forgive probably has to do with a Tribal issue of feeling betrayed or violated in some way (first chakra).

Now focus your attention on the items you have listed in the Tribal column. For each negative belief, relationship, or behavior pattern, describe what you think the Symbolic meaning might be. For example, the belief "I am always helping others who don't appreciate all that I do for them," taken Symbolically, represents your opportunity to understand the "rescuer" archetype in you—the need to heroically give yourself up to save another. Like many archetypes, the "rescuer" can be a positive role, but more often than not it leads to self-destructive behavior posing as altruism. At one time in human history, the rescuer was a genuine hero, yet the rescuing was generally done on behalf of the tribe and at the expense of the rescuer.

After identifying the Symbolic meaning, ask yourself, "What can I do to correct this behavior that would bring power and strength back into my system?" Then write down your answer in the Individual column. For example, "Before I offer to help someone, I will look more closely at my motivations for extending myself. If my motivation is to rescue or comfort someone, I will try to identify the reason I need to behave in this manner." You might ask yourself, "Did they ask for my help, or did I volunteer prematurely out of my need to make them need me?" Among couples, this kind of "altruism" may take the form of one partner "rescuing" the other, an alcoholic, in a way that enables the alcoholic partner to keep drinking. Or if your partner is describing a problem at work, you may jump in and offer ways to "fix" the problem, when all she wants is a sympathetic hearing. Your partner may even need to go it alone, and your attempt to "rescue" her may actually interfere with her process.

By utilizing these three distinct ways of viewing your beliefs and behaviors, you can learn to resolve problems and influence situations positively. By looking for the Symbolic meaning in a challenge, for instance, you are helping to detach your energy from the fear connected to that challenge. Symbolic perception allows you to create options for yourself that you would not otherwise have been able to conceive of within the limitations of Tribal sight. Introducing Symbolic perception into the Tribal realm, or into the day-to-day world in which you reside, helps you reorganize your physical environment according to a goal that connects the power of your body with your spirit. For instance, if you believe you are being punished for something you did wrong, replace it with the Symbolic perception "Every illness is an opportunity to learn something about myself."

Your Individual power then becomes the means through which you create a behavioral pattern focused intently enough to activate within your physical body the energy vibrating at the Symbolic level.

You can use these three forms of perception and power in every area of your life—to resolve problems, to understand conflicts in relationships, to appreciate the blessings that come into your life, and certainly to enhance your healing process. The Tribal column is your problem column; the Individual column is your activist column. Our Individual will and actions are what get us from the undifferentiated muddle of Tribal thinking into the world and then through the world to our spirits and healing. That is why taking action is so crucial to changing deep-seated negative beliefs and behavior and getting on with healing.

I realize that this is a complex procedure, so let's take one more example to make sure you've got it down. First, list a negative belief, relationship, or behavior in your Tribal column. An especially pungent example of a Tribal belief is that certain races, nationalities, or religions other than the ones into which you were born are inferior. We all fall prey to this form of belief in some way, yet these beliefs exist only at the external or physical level and have no meaning Symbolically.

Next, jump over to your Symbolic column and create a meaningful way of seeing that belief, relationship, or behavior so as to enhance your personal power.

One form of Symbolic thought is to see the problem in terms of some universal principle. In the case of a racist or nationalist belief, this can be as simple as saying, "All is one." Now in your Individual column, describe a course of behavior that would assist you in accomplishing the shift in consciousness from Tribal to Symbolic. If you are trying to effect a physical or psychological healing, you might write that you need to seek out a support group or therapist, or create a new inner discipline for yourself, such as keeping a journal in which you record all the things you are grateful for on each day of your life. Your aim here is to build a bridge between the Tribal column and the Symbolic column by committing to some personal action by which you can absorb into your physical system the positive energy released from the Symbolic level of reasoning. To return to the example of racist and nationalist beliefs, my best counsel would be to change your vocabulary: This is the active work to become aware of your perspective and change it. Watch how you say "we" instead of "I" in certain situations; be aware of your defensiveness toward others; start to challenge your identification with your nation or ethnic group. Begin to think of yourself, and speak of yourself, as a global being instead of an ethnic one. Is rising unemployment less of a problem in Japan than in the United States? Is ethnic conflict a dilemma only for African and Balkan nations?

Once you have a working grasp of Three-Column Sight, use the method on a regular basis to help you heal—it's a powerful tool. But it isn't meant to be used in isolation. I've listed a number of other useful ways to ignite your healing fire—a power that, once lighted, has no limitation. Use any or all of them in combination with Three-Column Sight to maximize your healing potential.

FUEL FOR THE FIRE

Learn to say no.

The most important thing you can do for yourself in a crisis situation is to learn to manage your time. You have to put yourself first on your agenda. The best way to do that is to learn to say no. You can no longer afford to live within the perception that you're going to miss out on something potentially life-changing if you're not there, whether the event is a new movie that everyone's going to see, or a family wedding, or a business meeting.

You have to remain focused on the fact that you are only here now, and you don't know what tomorrow will bring. The questions are essentially the same, whether you're completely healthy or are trying to heal: "Is this what I want to put my time into right now? Am I mismanaging the precious gift of time because I'm afraid I'll miss something?"

Any time you find yourself in a life crisis, ask the following questions:

1. Who are the most important people in my life?
2. Am I investing my time in the people and things that matter most to me, both for healing and for living a meaningful life?
3. If not, what am I willing to do about that?

Although these evaluative questions may seem more crucial during a transitional period—when you're having a healing crisis or a "spiritual emergency"—you should also be asking them on a regular basis throughout your life. As you need to conserve your energy and use it wisely, you have to learn to use your time wisely. You may need to cut down on the time you spend with people whose orientation and behavior no longer fits in with your need to heal. I'm not saying that if you're trying to heal cancer or a history of incest that you should spend time only with other cancer or incest survivors. But if there are certain people in your life—friends, family, or business associates—who talk and act in a negative way, who don't respect their own bodies, or who encourage you to behave in a way that doesn't facilitate healing, you need to ask yourself if you can afford to spend time with them. Just because someone wants you as a friend may not be a good enough reason to devote time to that person at this point in your life.

Nor am I saying that you have to be "doing something useful" at every moment, especially if "doing something" begins to take on a puritanical obsession with activity and productivity. Using time wisely means leaving empty space for yourself apparently to "do" nothing but actually so that you allow new ideas and feelings to come to the surface. This "inactivity" is the same principle behind meditation, only you can bring this quality of disengaging yourself from draining concerns and preoccupations throughout your day. In this sense, an illness, trauma, or life crisis can become an opportunity to explore your life at a slower pace. Saying no to doing something can mean saying no to making yourself busy just to be doing something. This principle can also be a useful counterbalance to the second way to ignite your healing fire.

Change course immediately.

Healing is a "present time" challenge. Many people begin their healing process by researching every possible form of treatment available. While they are doing this research, however, they are not actually doing anything about their condition. They are assuming that the knowledge they are pouring into their heads is, in itself, a healing force. People often comment to me that they are simply unsure of which treatment is best for them, and until they can figure that out, they feel "safer" not doing anything. I take that to mean that they are not ready to make the necessary changes in their lives.

Listening to the way they rationalize their inability to make a decision, I sometimes get the impression that standing still allows them—at least temporarily—to maintain the illusion that they are not really ill. They may prefer to believe they are in the midst of a bad dream from which they will eventually wake up. This phenomenon occurs most often in cases where people are not yet experiencing any physical pain with their illness.

Postponing the decision to shift gears is more than unwise; it is dangerous. It is much wiser, and safer, to start anywhere than to do nothing. Every positive choice is a good one and activates a new current of energy in your life. A new step or change does not have to be big to be effective. Along the way, continue to read up on all the information that expands your knowledge about what it takes to heal. Introducing a shift in your nutrition or adding an exercise regimen is a good beginning. You could start walking every day, or take a yoga class. If you can't locate a yoga teacher, purchase videotapes that offer instruction in yoga or other relaxation exercises. Read books about alternative health options, and try some of them immediately. If you feel you need group support, go to a holistic health resource center or health food store and check out the support groups in their listings or on the bulletin board. If you feel that a psychotherapist would be helpful, seek one out. You can make all these changes while you are in the process of seeking additional medical advice.

Above all, remind yourself as often as necessary that you can't afford to fall prey to the "I'll start tomorrow" way of thinking. There is only "now" in the healing process. Tomorrow, as they say, never really comes.

Practice cyclic thinking.

The perception that time and life are linear experiences handicaps the healing process. Examples: "If this treatment does not help within a month, it's not working and I must not be healing," and "At my age, what can you expect?" Your focus should be not on "time" but on the cycles of nature, which are mirrored in many other processes. In the natural world, seasons of warmth and ease and productivity are inevitably followed by periods of cold, difficulty, and retrenchment, but these difficult periods are themselves followed by a recurrence of warmth and pleasure. Few traditions understand this cyclic principle and flow better than the Chinese, whose spirituality, like that of Native Americans, is closely tied to the earth. As the *Tao Te Ching* (77) puts it:

The Way of Heaven is like the flexing of a bow.
The high it presses down; the low it presses up.
From those with a surplus it takes away; to those without
    enough it adds on.
Therefore the Way of Heaven—
Is to reduce the excessive and increase the insufficient.

                              (translated by Robert Henricks)

When you are in the winter of your illness, you may feel as if
the cycle will never come around to summer again, but that's when
it's essential to be disciplined in your thinking. Take a few minutes
to recall a previous time in your life when your fortunes seemed to
be at an especially low ebb. Evoke the way you felt then, paying
attention to the sensations in your body as you reexperience those
feelings of hopelessness. Then recall the turning point, and allow
yourself to feel your growing sense of relief and confidence as
things began to change in your favor. It doesn't have to be a major
event; it can be as simple as having been behind in a game that you
eventually won, or getting a letter of reconciliation from a friend
you thought you had alienated. The eventual outcome is less
important than the shifting tide of events. You may have lost the
next game; the friendship may finally have ended after all. And
someday you will breathe out and not breathe in again. But bear in
mind that healing is above all a learning experience, and one of its
biggest lessons is that life is characterized by impermanence and
flux. If you can learn to accept change with equanimity, you will
have mastered a lot more than just an illness.

Cyclic thinking is also one of the most effective means of
learning to forgive. Although it is difficult to release the need for
personal justice and for what you may feel is the appropriate rec-
ompense or punishment, from a Divine perspective, that is no more
your call to make than what you have coming for your own deeds.
At one of my workshops I met a very gentle and caring physician
who worked at a veterans' hospital attending to soldiers wounded
in combat. He felt that he was meant to do this work because from

childhood he had had dreams in which he was a soldier in the Civil War who killed relentlessly. His work became his means of balancing the killing in his "past life." Although he might have felt that he deserved to be punished for his lack of mercy, Divine justice chose instead to let him develop mercy in his current life.

When you are feeling overwhelmed by your inability to forgive some wrong or injury done to you, remind yourself of the ancient teachings about laws of karma that are echoed in Christian teachings: What goes around comes around—in this life or the next. It is not for you to decide the nature of justice on a personal level, which is just as well, since human justice is often much harsher and less well balanced than Divine justice. Your only task is to learn to forgive—and call back the energy you are wasting on events in the past.

Part of the problem with the victim mentality is that it overlooks the ways in which we ourselves perpetuate what was done to us. The next time you find yourself caught up in angry thoughts about a past injury, try this exercise in forgiveness. Look very closely at your actions over the past week and see if you are committing the same kind of injustice or abuse from which you suffered. It doesn't have to be anything dramatic. You may feel, for instance, that during your childhood you were wrongly judged by another person and that that has influenced how people think of you today. Even a simple act of being misunderstood by a parent or teacher at a crucial moment can continue to weigh on you. When you start feeling that weight, look at whether you have judged someone else in a similar fashion. At first, your judgment of another may seem inconsequential. You don't like the way a man dresses, so you judge that he's a slob. Maybe you then convert that judgment into gossip. Or you may comment on how a certain woman has achieved what she has in her career, implying that she lacks ethics or honesty. In that way, a seemingly innocent or minor judgment can have serious consequences. You need both to forgive yourself for making the judgment and to forgive the person who judged you unfairly all those years ago. It may help to recall the words of the Lord's Prayer: "Forgive us our trespasses, as we forgive those who trespass against us." To the extent that we forgive others, we are forgiven ourselves.

Have realistic goals for yourself.

Although all earthly things change, they do not necessarily change overnight. Many people who come to my workshops assume that they will master in one day intuitive skills that have taken me fifteen years to develop fully. Instant clairvoyance is possible, of course, but a more likely scenario is that you will develop your own intuitive abilities by paying careful attention to energy principles. Likewise, although it is possible that you may adopt a new point of view or new insights and heal in an instant, you will more likely need to work consciously with holistic teachings for a long time. Just as no one can learn to run a marathon in one day, living a healthy life or healing an illness requires that you practice regularly whatever healing disciplines you adopt, whether they are medical treatments, nutritional changes, an exercise regimen, visualizations, or meditation.

Many new fears emerge following the diagnosis of an illness, or when you encounter a setback on tragedy in your life. You need to be patient with yourself. If you feel depressed or anxious, try to step back and see when and in what context these feelings appear. They may reflect one of your negative Tribal beliefs. If so, use Three-Column Sight to try to see the greater symbolism or message behind the mood. You can also do the following exercise from the Sufi tradition, called "A Mile from Baghdad."

Close your eyes, and watch yourself walking down a lonely stretch of desert road that seems to go on forever—like a highway somewhere in the Middle East. Feel the sun beating down, the hot sand beneath your feet, an overpowering thirst and fatigue. Let yourself experience both the aridity of the place and your own loneliness and desperation. When those feelings begin to be palpable, find a modest outcropping of rock alongside the road and settle in for the night. Watch the sun set, and feel the cool night air come on. As you rest from your travels, breathe in the refreshing air and feel your body start to come back to life.

Now come out from the rock formation and look around. In the near distance, you can see a few twinkling lights, which are soon joined by others. They must have been there before, but in the bright desert sun you couldn't make them out. As you begin to hear soft strains of music, you realize that a city filled with people is actually quite close by, within easy walking distance. You believed you were in the middle of the barren desert, but you were really only a mile from Baghdad. Let the realization sink in that relief is near at hand, and you have only a short way to walk. As you relax in that knowledge, say a brief prayer of thanksgiving.

If you do not notice any change in your body in the first month of your effort to heal, it does not mean that changes are not happening. They are occurring on an energetic level, and they will eventually cause positive mental, spiritual, and even physical changes. You are a lot closer to your goal than you may realize.

During the healing process, confer with others who have experienced your illness. You can gain a lot of good information from those who are on the same path as you, but do not compare the course of your own healing to theirs. Remind yourself that what did not work for one person in the physical body may be exactly what you need energetically to begin to heal. Stay open to possibilities at all times.

Develop your willpower.

Desiring to heal is not the same as having the will to heal. Some people who want to heal may not have the will to make the life changes required in order for them to heal. You need to train your mind and emotions to respond to the positive commands you create. And these positive thoughts must become the dominant perceptions with which your mind and emotions connect. Doing a thirty-minute visualization once or twice a day and then returning to fear-filled thoughts the rest of the day negates the influence of your positive work.

Keeping your focus in a positive direction takes discipline, and that level of discipline requires practice. Think of how easily you are distracted when you attempt to keep your mind and emotions aligned to a single thought. Unless you are a practiced meditator, your mind will wander in every direction within seconds. I once led a group of students through an exercise in which I told them to choose a thought and lock their minds into that thought to the exclusion of any other. Within a moment or two, a number of students sat up and complained that the "noise" outside was interfering with the exercise or that the light was too bright to do any serious "inner work." Yet learning to detach from such distractions was precisely what they needed to learn.

Insisting that the external environment meet certain conditions before you are able to become internally focused is itself a distraction. You do not need to develop your focus as completely as a meditation master, but you do need to achieve a working relationship with your inner resources to be able to quickly eclipse a negative thought with a positive one and feel the positive energy that results. The use of a mantra—a phrase or word that you repeat silently to yourself—is very effective in learning to focus. The word or phrase can be the traditional Sanskrit "Om" or "Om Mani Padme Hum," from the Hindu and Buddhist traditions, or "Mother Mary" or "Jesus," or the name of a virtue such as "love" or "compassion," or any word or phrase that brings you peace, strength, relaxation, and quiet attention. You may also want to combine the mantra with deep, steady breathing.

Practice taking breath in slowly and evenly through your nose and pulling it down to your belly. Feel your stomach expand gradually as you breathe in—put your open palm against your navel at first so you can actually feel the expansion. Once your belly is full, continue breathing in, and this time fill your diaphragm—the middle area of your chest just above the stomach. If you still have the capacity, breathe in a bit more and fill your lungs and your upper chest. Hold this breath in for a few moments, and then gently let the air out through either your nose or your mouth. It may take some practice to develop the ability—and the lung capacity—to be able to breathe in this three-stage process, but the resulting sense of calm and equanimity is worth the effort. If you prefer, you can seek out a relaxation or meditation teacher to guide you through these and other simple practices. Books such as *Focusing* by Eugene Gendlin and *Are You Getting Enlightened or Losing Your Mind?: A Spiritual Program for Mental Fitness* by medical doctor Dennis Gersten give other inspiring, easy exercises for consistently substituting positive mind energy for negative thoughts. The important thing is to do your practices regularly and with discipline. Eventually they will become reflexive, and so will your physical energy's response.

Another way to learn to control your mind and emotions rather than be controlled by them is to practice with the distractions in your everyday life. For example, suppose you are having a conversation with someone who makes a comment that angers you. You immediately command your energy to be unresponsive to that comment. Or suppose you become irritated about waiting in traffic or impatient because a task is not working out the way you had intended. These are perfect situations in which you can practice commanding your energy to remain within your body instead of leaking out to situations that essentially have no meaning. You can even use techniques such as deep breathing or repeating a mantra to keep yourself centered in such situations. Keep your attention on the larger picture—your health—and remind yourself that compared with the recovery of your health, everything else is insignificant.

Healing is not a quest to solve your mysteries, but to learn how to live within them.

Life is full of mystery. In fact, life is only a mystery—a journey beset by fogs we didn't see coming and detours into magical gardens that we had no idea were being cultivated for us. Asking why the painful and wonderful events of our lives occur when and as they do is a useless waste of energy. We can never know all that was involved in creating these moments in our lives. In psychological—and Divine—parlance, these events are "overdetermined": So many factors, incidents, forces, and energies are involved in them that you can never determine any single cause.

Illness remains one of the leading mysteries in life. Why does it happen? "Why me? Did I do something to deserve it? Will I live through it?" You may wonder if this disease is tied to your traumatic marriage or your childhood or toxins in the environment. Get past the questions. Focus on your healing in the present time.

In your search for a reason for your illness or tragedy, no reply will be forthcoming. Turn yourself to the comfort of faith in Divine guidance. The purpose of the mysteries of our lives may well be to lead us out of our dependence on human reasoning and its limited ability to account for why things are the way they are and into the acceptance that Divine intelligence is actually in control of our lives. Divine intelligence works in ways that we cannot understand, yet we can come to understand that we cannot completely trust much else. Always remind yourself that you are living a mystery, not solving one. Live within the questions that you have, but do not allow them to take over your life, your thoughts, or your actions.

Practice letting go of your questions and placing them in the hands of the Divine. Visualize God or Buddha or Mary or Jesus or the Tao taking away your questions, taking them up into themselves, into their limitless energy, pulling them away from you and your energy. Feel yourself freed from concern and doubt and filled with a healing, gentle glow that suffuses every part of your body and mind. Know that you can see and feel this energy and glow at any time, that it is always there and available to you.

It's not always easy to keep faith. A gifted and loving minister once told me that offering comfort to the many people he cared for was much easier than his inner struggle with his own faith. His solution, however, was "to pray to a God I'm not even sure I believe in, because I have no other choice." He gave the same advice to parishioners who came to him in similar crises.

God hears every prayer, regardless of whether we believe in God at the moment we pray. The God or Divine Force for whom we are searching wants us to know how darkness feels so that when we make it to the light, we can tell others from our hearts the true meaning of the teaching, "Be not afraid, for I am with you always, even until the end of time."

Cultivate grace.

The teachings of all spiritual traditions inspire hope. They also allow us to glimpse the power and compassion of God and the dimension of miracles. Universal truths can help you see life as an eternal stream and an unlimited power.

When seeking to touch the energy of the Divine, we climb symbolically to the top of a mountain, like Abraham when he took Isaac to the top of Mount Moriah, Moses on Mount Sinai, or Jesus at his Transfiguration on Mount Tabor. The symbolic meaning of climbing a mountain is making a journey to see a world much greater than ourselves, and to see farther than we have ever seen before. At the top of the mountain, we ask, "Can I receive the full magnitude of the power within me? Can I hold on to the intensity of my focus and my vision of healing once I leave the mountain-top, where I glimpse the landscape of the soul and eternity?"

The spirit needs nourishment to heal, just as the mind and body do. Build up the courage to act by inspiring yourself with the stories and wisdom of those who have changed their lives for-ever through taking action, through entering the dark night of the soul fearlessly. Sample the wisdom of unfamiliar traditions: Read the tales of the Hasidim or explore the Kabbalah; entertain your-self with Sufi parables or the poetry of Rumi; study the sermons of the Buddha or the simple teachings of Thich Nhat Hahn; examine the writings of mystics from the Christian Desert Fathers to the Upanishad texts, many of which are surprisingly accessible.

These stories don't always make logical sense—in fact, they're probably more effective when they don't, because they have a beauty and an internal power that transcends rational thought. According to Buddhist tradition, Bodhidharma is credited with bringing the principles of Zen Buddhism from India to China. He is said to have sat in meditation in front of a wall for nine years, refusing to move. "I'm not turning around until somebody comes who really wants to learn what I have to teach," he said. One day a scholar named Hui-K'e approached Bodhidharma and, complaining that he had no peace of mind, asked how he could achieve it. The master put him off, saying that such an accomplishment would require arduous discipline and was not for the fainthearted. Hui-K'e, who had been standing outside in the snow for hours, again implored Bodhidharma for help and was again rebuffed. Desperate now, the scholar cut off his left hand and threw it in front of Bodhidharma, saying, "If you don't turn around, I shall cut off my head." Bodhidharma said, "You're the one I've been looking for," and accepted him as a student.

As you absorb truths and stories that nourish the spirit, you will feel an energy released within you. It is an energy that resonates with universal truth and leads you into unity with your world. This energy can only be called "grace." It is a vibrational force of such power that it can lift you for an instant out of your immediate circumstances. It can fill you with the perception that there is nothing you cannot handle and that all will be well, no matter the outcome. The Yehudi, a Hasidic rabbi who died in the early nineteenth century, told the story of a lifelong thief who in his old age was unable to ply his "trade" and was starving. A wealthy man, hearing of his distress, sent him food. Both the rich man and the thief died on the same day. The trial of the rich magnate occurred first in the Heavenly Court; he was found wanting and sentenced to Purgatory. As he approached the entrance to Purgatory, however, an angel came hurrying to recall him. He was brought back to the Court, where he learned that his sentence had been reversed. The thief whom he had aided on earth had stolen the list of his iniquities.

Grace is not always an obvious force, to be sure. It comes in many forms, some subtle and mundane, some powerful and transfiguring. Sometimes grace manifests as synchronicity—its energy brings together people or events in a soothing, helpful, or dramatic way when you most need it and least expect it. At other times grace is the energy that suddenly illuminates us with understanding, allowing us to see what we had not been able to grasp before. Grace can also lift us into an altered state of consciousness in which we feel suffused by an unfamiliar energy—an indescribable combination of love, hope, and fearlessness. Protective as well, grace can be a shield that surrounds us in situations that threaten us in some way: surviving a car crash that should have killed you, suddenly being overcome with a feeling that you need to return home, only to discover that you had left the stove on; meeting a "stranger" who offers you help just when you need it most. And grace does not work according to the laws of linear time; that's why an illness or a life crisis that should normally take years to cure or resolve can be healed in an unimaginably short time.

In case you think that miracles don't really happen to "ordinary" people or that all these stories are exaggerated, let me tell you a story that happened to me. Satya Sai Baba is a living saint of India who is said, among other things, to be able to manifest objects, from holy ashes to precious stones, out of thin air. This ability is known by the Sanskrit term *vibhuti*, which means "revelation" or "power." A few years ago at Findhorn I was having a lot of trouble keeping my balance. No matter what I did, the condition kept getting worse, so as a last resort before I went to sleep, I said a prayer to Sai Baba: "I need some *vibhuti*, and I need it now. I'm in bad trouble." The next morning I received a package from an acquaintance in Copenhagen whom I had met five years before and hadn't heard from since; inside was a small tube filled with ashes, with a label that read, "To Caroline Myss from Satya Sai Baba." Since the mail from Denmark to Scotland usually takes at least several days, the answer to my prayer must have been on the way to me before I uttered the words. I didn't know what to do with the ashes, so I took some out and, being an ex-Catholic, rubbed them on my forehead. Within hours of receiving the *vibhuti*, my balance returned, and I never had that problem again. I've since carried that tube of *vibhuti* with me wherever I go.

I have often been asked whether I believe that grace can actually save a person's life. There is no way to prove that it can, of course, but I choose to believe it can from the numberless reports of people who testify to the intervention of Divine energy in their own lives. One vivid story I was told was about a man named Steven, who had developed a serious case of internal and external hives, brought about from taking a new medication to which he did not know he was allergic. The rash began as a small irritation on his skin and proceeded to spread all over his body. After several days, Steven thought he must be allergic to something, but it never occurred to him that it was the medication. Instead, he reviewed the food he had been eating, the soap he was using, and the fabrics of the various items of clothing he was wearing. As the rash continued, Steven developed more symptoms. He broke into a fever every evening and became weaker by the day. He swelled up, retaining fluids in his tissues. Soon the fevers were constant and his weakness so severe that he could not walk. His feet were so swollen that he could no longer put on his shoes.

One morning, at the height of Steven's suffering, a voice woke him up and told him to get to a hospital because he was dying. Then the voice told him to breathe slowly and deeply, pulling his breath fully into his lungs. An image came into his mind of a yoga master leading him in this exercise. Steven was Christian, and although he was certainly familiar with yoga in an intellectual sense, he had never learned or practiced it. He phoned a friend, however, telling him that he needed to get to a hospital immediately. En route, he continued to breathe as instructed, and every time he closed his eyes, he saw the yoga master.

Steven arrived at the hospital nearly unconscious. He was rushed to the emergency room, where the attending physician immediately administered a shot of steroids. He informed Steven that he had developed a near-terminal case of internal and external hives, and that every organ in his body, along with his skin, was inflamed. He also informed Steven that if he had not arrived at the hospital within a few hours, he probably would have died.

"I had never given any serious thought to yoga, or to any teachings or practices from the Hindu tradition," Steven later said to me. "As far as I was concerned, yoga was nothing more than a physical exercise, hardly a spiritual practice. And I never thought of the breath as anything other than what we have to have to stay alive. Now I practice yoga constantly, though I no longer see that yoga master when I close my eyes. I have a 'normal' and physical teacher, but I still wonder each day, Why did a yogi come to me? I mean, I had no belief in that tradition at all. How did that happen? I'll never stop thinking about that experience. It changed my life—actually, it saved my life."

I realize that many people tend to be somewhat skeptical about stories like Steven's, and for a long time I felt that way myself. So many inexplicable occurrences have happened to me personally, however, that I have a hard time maintaining my skepticism. One of the most inexplicable involved a woman named Jenny, with whom I had been friends since high school. Jenny had become involved in a tumultuous relationship with Mark, a threatening and paranoid man who often exploded into episodes of screaming brought on by the slightest incident. He was a guard at a local prison. He kept weapons at home, and although he never actually threatened Jenny with a gun, he would glance at his weapons every time an argument erupted. By the time Jenny began to think about leaving Mark, she was so frightened of what he might do to her that she was unable to act on her instincts to get away from him.

When Jenny invited me over to meet Mark, I didn't know any of this about him, only that he was living with her. Almost from the moment I arrived, Mark and I had an intense clash of personalities. I thought it was humorous at first, because I had never gotten such a hostile reaction from anyone before. Another close friend of Jenny's was also there at the time, a woman named Barbara, who was a police officer. Barbara and I hit it off just fine, and for some reason I asked her for her phone number and address, even though

I wasn't expecting to contact her. As I was leaving that evening, Jenny and I embraced for a moment and I whispered to her, "We both need to pray to get you away from this guy."

I had such a gut feeling that Mark was psychotic that I phoned Jenny a few days later to tell her to get away from him. I also told her that I was keeping my promise to pray for her, and that I believed that she would be given the "grace" to leave Mark safely. Five days later, as I was going to bed, I had a strong visual image of Jenny being shot that night. I phoned her immediately, and when she answered the phone, I could hear Mark raging in the background, demanding that she hang up. Jenny managed to get out the words "Help me" before hanging up.

I immediately pulled out Barbara's phone number and called her. Barbara put out an emergency call to her fellow police officers, and together they arrived at Jenny's house. When no one answered the doorbell, they broke down the front door. They found Jenny on the floor in a corner, holding a chair in front of her for protection. Mark was waving his gun and threatening to kill her. Fortunately the officers were able to restrain Mark, who was arrested and jailed. Jenny packed her belongings immediately and left to stay with me for a while. She has since met another partner with whom she shares a loving and supportive bond.

We could say that the details of this experience—the timing of my meeting Mark, my request for Barbara's phone number, and the promise that Jenny and I made to each other to pray for the grace to resolve this situation—are nothing more than coincidences. But what makes the ingredients of a coincidence come together, after all? I personally believe that the energy of grace was behind this entire situation, if for no other reason than the manner in which the image of my dear friend getting shot entered into my mind that night. I knew instantly that I was receiving instructions to save Jenny, and I now know the feeling and power of the energy of grace.

Grace can also be thought of as the energy that comes over you like a soft blanket when you need comfort, filling you with the feeling that regardless of what roadblocks surround you, they will be removed when the time is right. Grace is an unreasonable force; it pays no mind to what we consider difficulties. It has the power to lift you beyond your abilities and to draw support into your life just when you need it. When such moments occur, ask yourself, as you give thanks for what you are receiving, whether the power behind the coming together of the right people or the right forces is the energy of grace. In all likelihood, it is.

Every situation in your life has been created with the energy of grace. Pay attention to the ordinary moments as much as to the extraordinary ones, and recognize that behind the scenes of those events is the energy of the Divine. Having faith in that which we actually experience is sometimes not nearly as challenging as having faith in a force we cannot see.

Use sacred imagery.

Several students have told me that learning to visualize the internal structure of their physical bodies is not nearly as difficult as learning to apply visualization to their energetic bodies. If you use the sacred imagery of the chakras, the Tree of Life, and the seven sacraments, however, your visualizations of spiritual energy may feel more tangible and effective. Because this process of visualizing the chakras is so complex yet so valuable, I will devote Chapters 7 and 8 to the chakras and the connection between them and the Christian sacraments.

But there are many ways to use sacred imagery. A recovering alcoholic named Gary came to me complaining that he kept slipping and returning to drink. He was a truck driver, and the long hours and travel left him with plenty of time and opportunity to go out drinking. "I just keep getting crucified," he said, in explaining that people's criticism of his drinking would then lead him to drink even more. It occurred to me to suggest using sacred imagery. I asked him if he identified with the Crucifixion, but he insisted that it was just a figure of speech. I discussed the archetypal meaning of the Crucifixion as a form of being scapegoated for the sins of others, as he no doubt saw happening to him. Then I asked him to image the cross with the chakras running from bottom to top along its vertical shaft, explaining that he could battle alcoholism by getting off the cross and allowing his alcoholism to be crucified instead of himself.

Gary responded profoundly to my suggestions. He did more than just visualize the cross with the chakras; he got a crucifix and put seven marks on it to represent the chakras. He wore it under his clothing, but at times he would take it out and touch, for instance, the first chakra at the foot of the cross and say, "This is the energy of the first chakra. I want to renew my life. I want to be rebaptized and to release the power of alcoholism." Touching the second chakra mark, he would picture himself having communion with God and accepting God's grace to get off this cross. In terms of the Tree of Life, he saw that communion as returning to him the male power and sense of manhood that he had lost through his alcoholism.

In Gary's case, he needed the physical object of the crucifix to touch; the visualization alone would not have been enough. And whenever he felt himself being tempted to slip, he would hold the crucifix and pray to refocus himself.

Whether you use visualization or actual objects, sacred imagery is a profound way to feel a connection with the heavens. The history of human spirituality is replete with images of the Divine and of all manner of saintly beings, angels, and spirits. Many Catholics, for example, believe that Saint Jude is the patron saint of "hopeless causes" and pray to him in difficult circumstances, such as apparently incurable physical illness. Miracles that have been credited to faith in a particular holy figure are not just pious folk tales—many of them have been authenticated by the most skeptical medical doctors.

Sacred imagery should be thought of as a way that our five senses can establish a tangible link to the Divine. Seeing or visualizing in some way is a basic human need, since we have difficulty relating to what we cannot perceive. Such a physical connection is not so much a matter of faith as a means of feeling an intimate bond with the Divine. Many of the world's Buddhists, who do not believe in a Supreme Being as such, nonetheless venerate images not only of the Buddha but of hundreds of different celestial and earthly bodhisattvas and of female spirits called *dakinis*. Jews and Muslims, whose religion forbids images of the Divine, use calligraphic renderings of sacred syllables and texts in Hebrew and Arabic to help focus their devotions. Given the vast size of the universe, you can derive great comfort from such a personal link to God, which reminds you that every prayer is heard and every thought is recorded.

If you have a favorite image of the Divine, a personal saint, or a revered spiritual teacher such as Ramana Maharshi, Pema Chodron, or the Dalai Lama, keep it with you. Although you can't carry around your altar or sacred space, you can carry a small image with you, reminding you that you are truly never alone. We need this level of comfort and confidence, not only to heal the body but to keep us centered whenever we feel ourselves slipping into the fears and anxieties generated by everyday life.

Learn something new every day.

There is great power in learning something new each day. Learning activates passion, and passion is power—in fact, passion is one of the strongest forms of energy that we can generate within our body. Passion is a connection to life itself, giving us a reason to want to see more of tomorrow.

A friend of mine developed a passion for cooking because he needed a special diet. Cooking also provided him with a reason to invite friends and family to his home on a regular basis. They came to see him celebrate the life he was creating in his kitchen, and he used the "creation" time he put into his meals as a healing metaphor for his body. A woman I know became an avid gardener because she loved growing plants that were life-sustaining and flowers that filled her home with soothing fragrances.

Like meditation, developing and pursuing a passion is its own reward, but it can generate many valuable "side effects" along the way. We can't even know where our passions will take us or what subsidiary benefits may accrue to us from following our hearts and our bliss. In a book called *Journey*, Robert and Suzanne Massie tell a dramatic story of raising their hemophiliac son, Bobby. As a young couple, the Massies had to educate themselves and their son about hemophilia, and also had to raise the consciousness of their family, their child's schoolteachers, and even health professionals about the condition. They courageously recount how they struggled constantly to provide the best, most informed care for their son throughout the late 1950s and into the early '70s when modern medicine was only beginning to understand how to treat the kinds of severe, painful, and life-threatening bleeding within joints and muscles that can occur in hemophilia.

As Bobby grew up, he was unable to roughhouse and play the usual childhood games because of the risk of serious injury. Often, Bobby needed casts on his limbs as a result of severe bleeds, and this further restricted his ability to interact freely and normally with other children. He would often miss weeks of school because of his bleeding and his need for special care, which put great demands on both parents and his siblings, isolating him and his parents in difficult ways.

Suzanne describes the pain she felt in watching Bobby's continuing ordeal as being almost unbearable, one factor that precipitated a spiritual crisis for her. She recounts a dark night of the soul in which she prayed for God's help and for strength to deal with Bobby's suffering. Eventually, through prayer and her determination to go on, she felt herself strengthened and learned a kind of patience in the face of her, Bobby's, and her family's destiny. Hers is a story of powerful compassion, rare insight, and profound spiritual growth.

One day, Bobby's knee became so badly swollen from bleeding in its joint, and the pain so excruciating, that he was delirious. Bobby was unable to tolerate even the weight of a bedsheet on his leg and could not bear to be touched. Suzanne kept vigil through the first day and night of Bobby's serious bleeding, through a second day and night, and on into a third. In the middle of that third night of her son's inescapable torment and her own fears for him, Suzanne felt an urge to do something different come to her clearly through her exhaustion. She decided to act on this strong urge and persuaded Bobby that he needed to move into a position that she somehow knew would ease his terrible pain. After resettling him, she placed pillows around his leg, and began to distract his mind from the pain by talking about the recent moon flight. In this way, mother and son broke for a few minutes the absolute hold that the pain had had over Bobby.

As Suzanne struggled to prepare Bobby for some desperately needed sleep, she prayed fiercely for help. She suddenly felt as if she had been ordered to put her hand on Bobby's knee. She argued with this impulse or directive, afraid to cause her son harm and further pain, but she felt clearly again that she was commanded to place her hand on his knee. Gradually, she moved her hand closer and closer, until she was lightly, touching his knee for a brief moment. Bobby was able to relax and sleep, and a welcome peace fell over Suzanne. She felt certain in her heart that the terrible episode was over.

In the face of her son's ongoing physical and emotional challenges, Suzanne needed to find something to engage her own mind, a mental challenge and discipline to focus her in another direction. She writes that an inner voice directed her to study Russian, to follow her passion for Russian music and dance. As she learned this new language, she also studied Russian history and read about the Romanovs, the last royal family to rule Russia before the revolution of 1917. Among their five children, the Romanovs had a son named Alexis, who also was a hemophiliac, although his condition was less severe than Bobby's. Robert Massie, then a journalist, had also become fascinated by the Romanovs and had written an article on Tsarevich Alexis. His fascination with Russian history and research into the Romanovs grew, until Suzanne suggested that he write a book on the subject.

As the years passed, Bobby learned to cope independently and positively with his condition. In a section of *Journey*, he writes that he learned much about himself because of his condition. The

Massies' own drive to learn about hemophilia led to their passion for Russian history and culture, which led to Robert's extensive research into the Romanov family and his writing of the best-selling book *Nicholas and Alexandra*, on which, he acknowledges, Suzanne was an invaluable collaborator. Robert writes that he and Suzanne had a strong sense of fate that as parents of a hemophiliac they would write a unique book, and its successful publication lifted the family out of difficult financial circumstances. Through meeting the challenge of Bobby's health, the Massies found their own gifts as writers, which became their gift to the world.

Remember, any passion will do. Find one. Follow one.

Create a new vocabulary for yourself.

I have already elaborated on the danger of living in the consciousness of woundology. Although there is no harm in expressing to another the pain and fear that illness brings into your life, you want to avoid falling into the pit of constantly "speaking pain."

Toward that end, create a new vocabulary for yourself that describes your condition in optimistic, healing, or spiritual terms. For example, refer to your illness as "a spiritual journey into a new part of yourself." One person I met referred to her illness as "a friend who has come to teach me great truths." Calling her illness a "friend" helped her lessen the fear of her situation because she never had a friend whom she feared. She associated her friends with love, joy, and trust, and by thinking of her illness as a friend, she felt that she could communicate with it. She felt it would leave her when their time together was complete, which is exactly what happened. Once healed, she actually held a ritual saying farewell to her friend—a fine antidote to lingering woundology that more people should try.

The purpose of creating a positive vocabulary for your situation is to assist you in "outgrowing your illness." You want to feel that you are larger and more powerful than the disease present in your body. You want to remind yourself constantly that you have numerous healthy resources in your body upon which you can rely to come to your assistance—you have love, you have hope, you have faith. These are powerful allies.

Try writing about your life as a journey, in a story entitled "My Biography Becomes My Biology." Write of all the wonderful experiences you have had in your life. Don't look for only the sad moments that could have contributed to your illness or life challenge. The positive times contribute to your health—use them. Write about the loving relationships you have now and have had in the past. Remember the fun times. Fill yourself with memories of times that made you feel in love with your life and grateful to be alive.

Ask the friends and loved ones in your support system to join you in creating a positive vocabulary for what you are experiencing. One man described his daily journey as "entering the well." Note that he established distance by using the word *the* instead of *my* when referring to the well. For him, this phrase held a profound double meaning: The well represented his daily effort to clear his emotions, and it also reminded him to keep his focus on getting "well."

Others have written poetic verses that they would repeat several times a day. Some even write verses to their favorite piece of music. You want to find the words that help you distance yourself from your illness and fill you with power. Remember, as you do this, to see yourself as larger than your illness and to become larger than the experience of illness. Think of your illness as no more than one or two words and then think of yourself as the editor of your illness who can rephrase and delete those words from your mind, your heart, and your spirit.

Review daily where you have plugged in your circuits.

Make it a daily practice to note where you have invested your energy. Pay attention to any feeling that energy is leaving your body, and assess why and where it is going. If your energy attaches itself to a target that is draining your energy, tell yourself to "detach." Learn to sense the flow of energy into and out of your body—all this requires is conscious attention. You already know the sensation of energy leaving your body when you are angry or frightened—you feel instantly weakened. Some people develop intense headaches or backaches. Interpret any physical symptom as a signal that you are losing energy.

As a preemptive action, direct your energy circuits each day into positive sources that can help you feel filled with power and light. One person I know visualized his circuits connecting to the statues of Jesus and Mary that stood in the church he attended. "Plugging into" those images every morning and evening made him feel consciously bonded to the energy of God. Other people I know have visualized their energy circuits connected to the power of the sun or other systems of nature that are endless in their life-force and that represent the ever-present support that nature provides for us.

Another effective means to connect or disconnect your circuits is to use your breathing. As you breathe in, imagine that you are retrieving your energy from whatever represents a drain on your system. You connect your energy by inhaling, breathing in your own energy and power. Visualize a symbol of strength and power as you get ready to exhale. Focus on your symbol, exhale, and release your energy with the words "I am merging with the energy of this symbol of strength and power. I ask that its energy flow into my system constantly." Once you have connected to a symbol that represents power for you, its energy flows into you constantly.

Practice gratitude whenever you feel overwhelmed.

You may easily feel confused by a sea of suggestions for your healing. By the time you get through all of your meditation practices, therapeutic work, and daily exercise, it may appear that you have run out of energy and daylight. In truth, it need not be as overwhelming as it looks.

Positive attitudes, along with Three-Column Sight, eventually become a habit and not an effort. By eating a proper diet, you are still eating several times a day; the only difference is in what you are eating. Keeping a journal may be a new practice in your life, so do it once a week, and if you come genuinely to enjoy it, do it more often. Most of all, try as much as possible not to fear your illness but to find ways to stay inspired.

Few practices soothe our spirits as much as gratitude. Feeling appreciative of all that life has given us and continues to give us makes life thrive in our systems. Make gratitude a practice. Do not look for only the large and obvious as a reason for gratefulness. Learn to see your life through a wide-angle lens that includes every detail.

Finally, in your effort to appreciate all that is in your life, include yourself. Spoil yourself with gifts of time—time to know yourself better and time to love and appreciate those who are a part of your life. Or just plain indulge yourself in ways you have always wanted to but for which you never gave yourself permission. Wander off your beaten path.

Healing is, admittedly, a lonely journey. Few obstacles that we will ever encounter are life-threatening, but disease is. Psychologically and spiritually devastating experiences like the loss of a child or a painful divorce can be just as dangerous; the anguish they generate can in some cases lead to a large-scale physical breakdown or even suicide. Be committed to your effort to return to mental and physical health. Don't let the limitations that you experience today influence what you may experience tomorrow.

All things are possible, and heaven is always listening.

Chapter Seven

VISUALIZING
THE CHAKRAS

As we have seen, the physical body has seven levels of internal power. Each level of power is not only aligned to a physical system within the body but also relates to external and internal issues that are part of our lives. This view of the body is actually quite ancient. The teachings and the scriptures from the Buddhist, Hindu, Hebrew, and Christian spiritual traditions all make reference to the seven sacred levels of power that contain and manage the life-force that flows through the body. The symbolism of the chakras, the Tree of Life of the Jewish Kabbalah, and the seven Christian sacraments represents an internal road map, a spiritual maturation process that can lead us from the unconscious to the conscious mind, then on to the superconscious.

The seven levels of our energy body record the most minuscule details of our lives and how we distribute our life-force. This intimate record-keeping is meant to assist us in investing our life-force consciously, in using our energy in ways that feed the spirit instead of weakening it. We develop spiritually by learning the lessons of each level of power and developing ever more sophisticated qualities of self-understanding and discernment.

One good way to become familiar with these seven levels of power is to practice actively visualizing the energy of each of the chakras. The visualizations in this chapter may help you connect with your seven power centers and make these energies more real and useful to you. They use not only the Eastern imagery of the chakras but the more familiar Western imagery of the Christian sacraments, as well as the sefirot of the Tree of Life in the Jewish Kabbalistic tradition. You can envision the chakras, the sacraments, and the sefirot working together to create the energy of a healing fire.

In all spiritual traditions, fire is a force that can purify the body. It burns away illness, corruption, and negative influences. Using the image of the healing fire and your own imaging abilities, you can catalyze healing at all levels of your being—physical, emotional, and spiritual.

In visualizing the merger of the chakras, the sacraments, and the Tree of Life, be aware that you may not always be able to come up with clear images or with any images at all. Sometimes your visualizations may seem vague or elusive. That's all right: The most important element of this work is to do it in a disciplined way and to incorporate into that discipline a faith and trust that it is genuinely effective. Attempt to give form to the invisible, and trust that the invisible world works with the physical. Making visualization a natural, habitual part of your consciousness will allow the healing fire to work within you even when you're not thinking about it. Once ignited, that fire becomes part of your unconscious. It emerges in your dreams and intuitions and infuses you with a vital power.

You may want to tape-record the visualizations that follow the discussion of each chakra. Then you can play them back and follow them with your eyes closed, without losing focus on your internal energies.

THE FIRST CHAKRA

The first chakra is the Tribal center of our bodies. Within the Hindu tradition, it is called Muladhara, which in Sanskrit means "root support." Buddhism recognizes this center as an earth point of connection. Through this chakra, at the base of the spine, flow the roots of the Kabbalistic Tree of Life, referred to in Hebrew as Shekhinah. And within the Christian tradition, this center is symbolically represented as the sacrament of Baptism. Though each of these traditions uses different words to refer to the power of this center, they are all referring to the same quality of energy, which is considered to be feminine, symbolic of the earth. If you can think of all the different ways to describe this energy as one united force, you can begin to grasp the nature of the power of the first chakra.

The energy of our first chakra is meant to ground us, to make us feel that we are a part of the grand universe of life but also inextricably connected to the physical dimension of life. Because this energy is so directly rooted in physical life, because it nurtures and is nurtured by connection, it is considered a feminine force. This force can be thought of as our link to the actual energy of the earth itself. A strong and positive connection to this chakra's energy is essential to our health because we are energy beings. Our physical body produces and thrives on electrical currents that, in turn, connect us to the physical life patterns of the earth.

When we do not acknowledge this connection or when we otherwise violate it, we experience the shadow side of the first chakra. We become unbalanced; we have difficulty manifesting in the physical world; we cannot make things happen as we would like them to; our creative efforts are blocked and frustrated. Every life-form requires some degree of connection to the magnetic field of the earth. If we short-circuit our own vital connection, we cannot run the energy through our own systems that is necessary for us to be effective in the world, to perform acts of physical connection and creation.

Another aspect of the shadow side of the first chakra is an inability to find a place on the earth that "feels like home." Those who lack a conscious connection with the first chakra often find that many places to which they travel are beautiful, but none seems to lock into their system in such a way that they feel called to live there. They long for a place to reside and for a community to which to belong; even though they may ultimately choose to make an area their home, something about their connection to that place always seems incomplete.

Illness, too, often produces the sensation that we are losing touch with our physical world, that we have separated ourselves from the most intimate part of our personal lives. From the point of view of energy medicine, that sensation represents the disconnection of energy from the roots of life, or the first chakra. This disconnection leaves you with a somewhat "drifty" perception of the world around you. Your passion for the sources of joy that fill your physical environment may lessen. You may feel isolated and lost. But by focusing on the energy of your root chakra, you can reconnect to your energy and reverse its flow back into your life.

The First Chakra: Igniting the Fire

Focus on Shekhinah—the feminine creative energy in your life—and Muladhara, the root of your life. Visualize what these roots are; see what animates you, what your roots are actively embedded in; what gives you nourishment and nurture. Visualize your energy circuits making contact with everything that is significant and precious to you within your physical environment: your home or residence, your life partner, friends, or close family members; your work; your favorite possessions or avocations. Feel that connection with all your senses; direct your energy to extend out from your system to connect with and be recharged by everything that you are holding in your mind and heart. Feel yourself filled with the strength of all of these positive forces, these energetic riches.

Now, shift your attention to the symbolic meaning of the sacrament of Baptism—the celebration of accepting with gratitude every aspect of your life and all those who are a part of your life. Think of yourself as being reborn into your own life, contributing your vital life-force to the whole of your life. Feel that life-force returning to you while repeating, "I connect to all that is in my life. I am filled with the energy of gratitude, and I am allowing that energy to flow with all its strength through my physical and spiritual body."

THE SECOND CHAKRA

Your second chakra or energy center is known as Svadisthana, meaning "creative feminine abode," in the Hindu tradition, and Yesod in the Hebrew tradition. In the Christian tradition, it represents the sacrament of Communion. In the Kabbalistic tradition this center is generally considered to be male, symbolic of the active physical energy essential for creation. But it can also be feminine because it is the center of the creation of life, and both masculine and feminine energies are required for the creation of physical life. You both give and receive tangible life-force from the second chakra, leaving and entering through your sexuality. It is centered in the sexual areas of the body.

Like the first chakra, this energy center is a magnetic stronghold. Instead of keeping us rooted to our tribes, however, it serves to attract others to us and us to them. We relate one-to-one with this energy, finding partners and mates as well as adversaries. The second chakra is the core of our instinctual nature. It activates our sexual desires, alerts us to dangers we cannot physically see and, when necessary, provides us with a degree of physical strength that exceeds our normal requirements. For these reasons, the second chakra can be thought of as our survival center. It generates physical life and protects it.

The shadow side of the second chakra develops when we immerse ourselves in feelings of aggression, hostility, vengeance, or greed, or when we dwell continually on memories of betrayal, physical violence, or sexual abuse. This state of mind can produce several dysfunctions, including impotence—both sexual impotence and the inability to generate the magnetics of creativity in one-to-one relationships. We may become unable to maintain a vibrational link to those with whom we have personal relationships, because our energy is being drained faster than it can be replenished, a consequence of our obsession with negative thoughts.

The Second Chakra: Igniting the Fire

Focus first on the energy of Yesod, on your sense of creative strength. Bring into your mind, heart, and spirit images of what you have created in your life, and then generate images of what you would still like to create. Visualize circuits of your energy flowing from your second chakra into the images of all that you desire to create, seeing life emanating from your energetic body, and then focus on the nature of Svadisthana. As you do this visualization, repeat the phrase "I am a vessel of creation. I am magnetically alive, and I am able to create life."

Now focus on the sacrament of Communion, representing your link to the many relationships in your life. Communion symbolizes the perception that each person in your life, regardless of the quality of your relationship, plays a Divinely ordered role. Center your attention on the relationships you view as negative, and imagine yourself unplugging your energy circuits from them. Don't allow your inability to understand how the person might have contributed anything positive to your life be a deterrent; work at this no matter how difficult you find it, until you can do it with ease and in genuine gratitude. Tell each person that you are grateful for the role they played in your life and yours in theirs. Then feel or image your energy circuits returning to your system and sealing your second chakra, so that no more energy is lost.

When that part of the exercise is complete, focus your attention on the loving relationships in your life, and allow that love to fill your second chakra with a glowing yellow light. Direct your energy circuits to these people, sending them your love and imagining a union between you and them. Once again repeat the phrase, "I am a vessel of creation. I am magnetically alive, and I am able to create life." This is the deepest symbolic meaning of the sacrament of Communion.

THE THIRD CHAKRA

Within the Hebrew tradition, the third energy center contains two forces intensely vital to our spirits—Hod, representing integrity and majesty; and Nezah, symbolic of the capacity to endure. In the Hindu tradition, this energy is presented as Manipura, meaning the "city of the shining jewel," and in the Christian tradition, it relates to the sacrament of Confirmation. All of these descriptions refer to the same essential spiritual powers: self-esteem, self-respect, and integrity.

Respect for ourselves is necessary to healing. A lack of self-respect, or a dishonorable character, is itself an illness. When we lack the fundamental spiritual qualities of endurance, integrity, honor, and self-esteem, healing the physical body becomes a double challenge.

You can easily sense when you are entering the shadow side of the third chakra: it manifests as shame, inadequacy, self-consciousness, and fear of others. Negative feelings drain the energy you need to heal. Reflect on what undermines your endurance and integrity, on where your energy leaks occur. Integrity is not solely the manner in which you conduct yourself with others. Think of it as the manner in which you conduct yourself with yourself. Can you make a commitment to yourself and keep it with integrity? Can you promise yourself to change your personal behavioral patterns (a discipline associated with the third chakra) and then keep that promise? To build endurance, can you commit to a shift of lifestyle and withstand the discomfort of walking that new path? Can you look at yourself and feel proud of your own honor code?

While all of the chakras play a vital role in your healing, the third chakra contains the energy of endurance—the power to endure the journey. The commitment to yourself to go the distance can be considered the backbone of your healing challenge.

Your commitment to yourself gives you the capacity to endure what may seem psychologically, emotionally, and physically beyond your limits. As a matter of spiritual honor and self-respect, your commitment to heal reflects your regard for the sanctity of your own life. Maintaining this commitment—day by day and hour by hour, actively and passively, in your dreams and in your thoughts—generates an intensity of self-esteem and self-awareness.

The Third Chakra: Igniting the Fire

Reflect on what you need to do to heal physically, emotionally, and spiritually. Bring your attention to your center chakra. Feel the messages that it sends you. What do you need to let go of? What do you need to keep? How will letting go or hanging on affect your healing?

Vow to do all that you need for your physical, emotional, and psychological body. The most significant promises are the ones you make to your own spirit. Your spirit needs hope, inspiration, prayer, and the energy of forgiveness. Promise your spirit that you will live in present time and so nourish it and yourself. Pray each day. As you pray, retrieve your spirit from your past. Leave behind memories and places you should have left behind long ago, even if the "long ago" occurred as recently as today.

Put your vow to heal in both general and specific terms, and write it down to help you realize all that you need to do for yourself:

"I promise to live and be in present time at all times. This means that I will put aside words and issues between me and my partner, or me and my children. I will stop working myself too hard and make time for my exercise and new nutritional regimen. I will meditate twice a day and practice right speech and right action with myself and others." Think of all that you want to do and must do to heal.

When you work on writing your vow, you may find it empowering to think of it exactly as the Hindu tradition describes the third chakra, as a "city of the shining jewel." Imagine that each promise you make is a jewel in a crown, and that the crown represents the essence of divine power, drawing that life-force directly into your spirit and body. Because it is difficult to maintain a commitment of this magnitude, it may help you to carry a copy of the written vow with you, if only to touch it and remind yourself to stay in the moment whenever you feel yourself slipping. At such times, you can also repeat this invocation: "I am filled with the energy of endurance and honor. My thoughts and words carry the power of creation itself." And always remember that your commitment, when truly made with integrity, constantly transfers power to you, even if you are not conscious of it.

THE FOURTH CHAKRA

The Hebrew term for the fourth energy center is Tif'eret, symbolic of the energy of harmony and beauty. Its Hindu name is Anahata, meaning "not stuck" (flowing with the pure energy of creation). In the Christian tradition, this center is aligned with the sacrament of Marriage, which of course is symbolic of the marriage to another person but is also symbolic of an internal union of body, mind, and spirit within the individual. This is the middle energy center, and it mediates between the lower three and the upper three chakras. It is through the heart that the mind is meant to channel the actions it supervises, and it is the heart that mediates with compassion and discernment the basic, instinctual feelings, energies, and actions governed by the more physically oriented chakras. The energy of the heart center also lifts us from the physical world and brings us more directly into contact with our internal world, especially with the ways in which we understand love.

It is almost impossible to mistake the energy of real love, our purest connection to the life-force. It is the most powerful force that runs through us. We all recognize when we feel unloved, whether we have lost someone we love or recognize that a relationship is not fulfilling us. This lack causes an excruciating drain on our energy system.

Self-serving love and possessiveness also drain our energy. When we love anyone or anything conditionally, we interfere with the free flow of this precious emotion contained in the symbolic meaning of Anahata, "not stuck." The shadow side of love and its energy manifests as bitterness, jealousy, and lack of forgiveness. These shadow emotions also interfere with our ability to love and respect ourselves. They prevent us from a symbolic marriage of our inner energies and from vowing to love, honor, and protect our emotional energy.

Healing demands the energy of love, especially love and care for yourself. Healing also benefits from the power of the love of life, nature, your own creativity, and love of the Divine. Admittedly, you cannot force yourself to fall in love with someone or something; nor can you make a person just show up in your life because you need that energy. But you can pray for Divine love, for help in opening your heart to others, and for the compassion to treat yourself with gentleness.

You can also develop a personal ritual in which you take yourself into your own heart. Do something enjoyable or appreciative each day for yourself. Use meditation tapes, soft music, yoga, or massage to assist you in feeling tranquil so that a sense of harmony can penetrate into your spirit and your physical body. If you need the assistance of a therapeutic or spiritual guide, by all means seek one out.

The Fourth Chakra: Igniting the Fire

There is always a path to the self. Begin by doing something for your-self that you have always wanted to do but have postponed, for what-ever reasons. Read poetry that brings you strength and inspiration. Take up drawing or painting or sculpting or playing a musical instru-ment or carving or dancing. Listen to music that makes you feel peaceful. Take a trip to a place you've never gotten around to visiting. Get the pet you always wanted but never took time for. Acting on a true desire always gives back energy and love to you.

Loving other people gives you energy that is healing, so take time to celebrate with those people you love the fact that they are in your life and you are in theirs. Let them know how much you mean to them. Be conscious of your own gratitude for the love that is in your life—it truly is a gift that is both given and received.

When you need to connect with a Higher Energy, practice the following visualization:

See or feel yourself connected to Divine energy, and imagine that energy flowing back through your connection into your system. Release into that energy your needs and fears. See that energy return-ing to the heavens, like a letter that has been sent and received by a friend. See your body and your life as one spiritual entity.

Now visualize circuits of your energy transferring messages of love to all the people you cherish in your life, and feel the energy of their love return to your system. Now, visualize your energy carrying messages of love into the world around you, connecting with the energy of nature and all of life. Picture yourself as large as the galaxy and capable of encompassing in your heart the Divine energy that exists at the root of all creation. Feel yourself vibrate in sync with that energy. See and feel yourself become one with this energy, which is the life-force itself.

The free-flowing, "nonstuck" life-energy of Anahata reminds us that love is a purifying force. Love gives us the power to clear away the weight of past emotions. See and feel this vital force overriding any diversions of your life-energy into past events. Feel the weight drop from your mind and body. Visualize your emotional burdens rushing out of your system, like debris in a stream of water. With your purified vision, you can now see and appreciate all that is in your life, even your history that has brought you to your present moment. Feel the soothing effect of this cleansing. Now see this soothing energy as your favorite symbol of harmony and inner tranquillity. As you do this visualization, repeat to yourself, "I ask the Divine to fill my body and spirit with the healing power of love strong enough that I can feel its power. I need this power so that I may heal and live a full life."

THE FIFTH CHAKRA

In the Hindu tradition, the fifth center contributes the energy of Vishuddha, meaning "purified." This fifth chakra combines physical and spiritual energies. Through a pure use of will, we act toward others in ways that transmit our strength of spirit. The Christian counterpart is the sacrament of Confession, which purifies our mistakes by urging us to acknowledge them openly, with neither guilt nor denial. In Buddhism, the fifth chakra represents "right speech," again referring to our capacity to speak honestly. This chakra contains the energy of the Hebrew forces of Hesed and Gevurah. The former represents greatness and love, our capacity to speak honestly to others and about others, and our respect for the power of truth. Gevurah is symbolic of right judgment, and its energy thrives when we exercise a compassionate discrimination and do not misuse our power to judge others harshly and unfairly.

Right speech and honesty inspire others and enhance our own energy systems. Conversely, we lose substantial amounts of power through the careless use of our will, especially when we act in the thrall of misperceptions and unfair judgments. You can sense

the energy of a negative and costly judgment because instanta-
neously you feel that you have made a mistake. Your energy flows
from your system like fluid draining out of a broken glass. This
drain also occurs when you make negative judgments about yourself and your own behavior. And any defensiveness about your
misjudgments of others increases your energy loss. Dishonesty, a
shadow aspect of the fifth chakra, creates more energetic exhaustion because you have to "protect the lie" you've created. Such
negative mental attitudes trigger an adrenaline reaction in the
physical body and frequently result in chronic exhaustion, depression, and low self-esteem.

These negative attitudes and judgments are acts of dishonor
to your life-force. The energy they create is repaired only by an
act of honest retrieval. This is where the strength of the Christian
sacrament of Confession comes in. Confession is the means
through which we retrieve the energy of our misjudgments and
lies. It is essential to your healing to make right those mental or
verbal thoughts that you have generated through the misuse of
your willpower. To make a Confession, you can turn to a spiritual
guide, such as a priest or a rabbi. Or you can seek out someone
who represents to you a higher level of spiritual maturity or moral
authority and who can serve as a witness. Completing a Confession, as humbling as it might be in the beginning, will give you an
exquisite sense of lightness. Seek the company of a trustworthy
person to whom you can unburden your spirit.

The Fifth Chakra: Igniting the Fire

Confess to yourself the troubles you have caused yourself and others.
Be specific. By admitting to such actions, you empty yourself of the
toxins generated by the shadow side of your willpower. As implied
in the Sanskrit meaning of this energy center, you must purify your
will and intentions as part of your spiritual journey. Strive to make
your intentions and will clean. The energy of all that you do to

heal, including your visualizations, will become more powerful as a result. A contaminated will contributes only a contaminated energy. Remind yourself of that truth as you do the visualization exercise that follows.

To help your self-confessions, you might want to write down on a piece of paper your misdeeds and misjudgments and then burn it. This ritual holds a great deal of healing power, but it is not quite as powerful or purging as confessing to another person who represents the energy of forgiveness. We all need to perform some type of a confession ritual, regardless of whether we are presently coping with an illness. The energy that is returned to you upon its completion is profound and immediately tangible to your spirit and your physical body.

To purify oneself is a sacred act, not an exercise in humiliation. Hold in your mind at all times that from a sacred perspective, confession is among the most honorable acts any human being can perform, precisely because it releases the weight of shame and so makes room in the spirit for the energy of pure judgment and truth.

Part II

Close your eyes, and imagine the people with whom you have "fifth chakra unfinished business." To whom do you need to say something to retrieve your spirit? Who continues to mystify you or trouble you? Relationships *are* mysteries, from how they show up in our lives to why they are there at all. Think of them symbolically. How have these people served a positive role in your life?

Invite the energies of Gevurah (right judgment) and Hesed (the power of unconditional love and gratitude) to come alive within you. See these energies around you and the people whom you are visualizing.

Acknowledge that you have no idea of the spiritual reasons these people are or were in your life; for all you know, they may have been the perfect catalyst that triggered a success. Imagine yourself in a symbolic dialogue with them. Express gratitude for the role they have played in your life and for your opportunity to be in theirs. With each person you think of, repeat the phrase "I hold you in gratitude, and I withdraw every circuit of my energy from all that I have judged."

As difficult as this exercise may seem at first, remind yourself of the many times you have been misjudged by others—it will recall the pain of that feeling into your system. Then focus your attention on those whom you have misjudged, and hold them in compassion. See your anger toward those who have misjudged you as a cloud apart from you. Allow it to float far away. Draw into your every breath the energy of forgiveness.

THE SIXTH CHAKRA

The symbolism of the sixth chakra is revealed in the Hindu word Ajna, Sanskrit for "command." Ajna represents the ability to see clearly and compassionately and is also symbolized by a third eye. The Kabbalistic counterpart is the pairing of Binah, which merges the limited power of human reasoning with Divine insight, and Hokhmah, which symbolizes our capacity to invoke the power of Divine wisdom to guide our perspectives. On the symbolic level of insight, the Christian sacrament of Ordination tells us that we each play a significant role in the evolution of life on this earth, regardless of how that role manifests on the physical plane. If our occupation seems insignificant from the social point of view, we may decide erroneously that we are insignificant from the spiritual point of view. Yet each part of our lives is valuable to our life as a whole and to the universe as a whole. Symbolically, we are each meant to respond to a call to service. We need to ordain ourselves and accept that our lives are meaningful, even if we can never know what our overall contribution is.

The shadow side of the sixth chakra is self-doubt and the detrimental practice of comparing ourselves to others. When we lose sight of our own self-worth, we become unbalanced and regard others with hostility, envy, and negative judgments. These emotions threaten our health, and we get a feeling of "going nowhere." We blind ourselves to all that we can contribute to the lives of others, and we lose our symbolic sight. The following visualization exercise can help you regain your balance and Symbolic sight.

The Sixth Chakra: Igniting the Fire

Visualize the energies of Binah and Hokhmah as Divine understanding and Divine reasoning. Imagine that you have been lifted above the limited view of your life and can see the whole of your life through a Divine lens. Use this larger perspective to encompass the symbolic meaning of the sacrament of Ordination, the truth that your life has purpose and meaning far beyond what you can comprehend. From this vantage point, invite the power of Divine reasoning into your system. Do not expect a verbal response to your request; expect an energetic one, a feeling of clarity and direction. Repeat to yourself the mantra "I welcome the energy of Divine wisdom and Divine reasoning into my spirit, and I release the judgments I have made about the value of my own life and the lives of other people. I accept the sacredness of my life, and I believe that my life is of service to this Universe."

Connect with the energy of Ajna with the invocation "I accept that Divine reasoning has precedence over any and all views that I might create in my own mind." Let go of your own views and values, and allow the unknown wisdom of the Divine—which feels like empty space—to enter your consciousness. Imagine an empty room; imagine a sunset; imagine a full moon; imagine the endless sea; imagine a star-filled night sky—any image that will clear out the mundane thoughts from your consciousness to leave space for something more inspiring. Feel yourself expanding to the size of that space, and breathe that "size" into your system while repeating, "I release the limitations of human reasoning toward others and toward myself. I live in trust and I have no more questions." Know that you have dissolved any judgments that weaken your spirit.

THE SEVENTH CHAKRA

The energy of the seventh chakra is our purest connection to Divinity. It is reflected in the Hindu symbol of Sahasrara, meaning the "thousand-petaled lotus" of enlightenment, or the Divine in every thing. In Buddhist teaching, the seventh Lotus represents that the Divine is eternal, ever-compassionate, and always present. This energy corresponds to the Hebrew symbol of Keter, the indescribable nature of God. It also corresponds to the Christian last sacrament, Extreme Unction, symbolic of the release of all that is "dead and over" in our lives. Together, these forces can be transformative and help us reach a level of perception that allows us consciously to experience the Divine and the energy of grace.

When you reach this point of power in your meditative practice of visualizing the seven chakras, you can understand the truth in the teaching "There is nothing else—only this." Take a minute to reflect on the clarity you have reached after letting go of the spiritual and physical debris of your life. You do not have to feel that you have "completed" the meditative exercises of all the other chakras to tap into this energy. The energy of this chakra flows into your being with or without your awareness of it, but when you pray to receive it, you can direct it to change your life. The energy of the seventh chakra dissolves fear, opens your heart completely, releases the limitations of your mind, and assists you in blessing the whole of your life. It helps you connect and communicate with the energy of God.

The shadow side of this chakra's energy is lack of faith and trust in the Divine and fear about any aspect of our lives, from what will become of us tomorrow to the closure of our lives on this earth. Nothing feels secure to us because our sense of safety is rooted in externalities and the physical world. We hold on to our pasts, which continue to affect our lives adversely. Because we are looking backward, we do not appreciate the grace and guidance that pour into our lives each moment, and we cannot see the fullness of each moment. Releasing ourselves from our past and absorbing the precious healing force that accompanies the "here and now" is the way in which we open ourselves to this energy, which represents the purest manifestation of the life-force.

Of all the chakras, this one may require the least amount of "conscious" effort to activate. Any and all prayer opens our seventh chakra. Like the Buddhist image of the lotus, which bursts into glorious bloom from out of the muck of swamps, it expands into full bloom of its own.

The Seventh Chakra: Igniting the Fire

Enter the energy of the seventh chakra by visualizing yourself unplugging your circuits from all that you no longer need to carry. Let go of the emotions and psychological weight of your own history. Let go of all the worries and stress that you are carrying for others. Into the space left by these worries, visualize the bright energy of union with the Divine in your body and spirit. Feel and see yourself healing.

Focus your attention on the energies of Keter and Sahasrara, which represent the intimate bond between you and God. Repeat to yourself, "I have no focus, I have no questions. I empty myself of all weights and worries. I am union." Let your thinking mind go to sleep as you enter a state of mindlessness and oneness.

Feel the energy that flows from your crown into the center of your body, to your root chakra and back up. It penetrates you with inexplicable, indescribable spiritual beneficence. It is your right. Simply request it. It is your own life-force, the part of you that connects to the formless, impersonal Absolute. The energy of the seventh chakra is the part of you that makes you know you are larger than your individual life. Feel how even a moment's contact with this energy can entirely reshape the way you handle your personal life.

THE EIGHTH CHAKRA

The eighth chakra is the most intriguing for me by far. I introduce this chakra apart from the other seven because it represents our next level of evolution. As such, it does not influence our physical bodies nor our personal, emotional and psychological nature as directly. The eighth chakra contains our archetypal patterns, the universally recognized themes or images that provide an impersonal, symbolic view of our human experiences. This dimension of consciousness connects us with others in an impersonal experience of human evolution.

It represents a warehouse of the kind of universal information and consciousness to which we will gain access as we enter the Aquarian age. This chakra is the connective link or bridge between our personal consciousness and the impersonal, greater consciousness of the archetypal dimension. While it does not have a counterpart within our bodies, as the other seven chakras do, it is located atop the energy field that surrounds and permeates the body and connects most immediately with the seventh chakra of insight.

As we move into the Aquarian age, the archetypes are going to become more apparent in us and accessible to us. As they do, the eighth chakra will take on even greater importance. This chakra has always been there, but we have not been able to gain access to it until recently. Just as we can now see ultraviolet light with the aid of electronic equipment, we have been developing the meditative, conscious ability to see beyond the visible world and perceive the energy dimension of our lives. As human consciousness evolves, we become more sensitive to an increasingly refined vibrational field.

I began to sense the energy from the eighth chakra in 1990, as I was doing a reading on a woman with chronic fatigue syndrome. Unlike all of the previous readings I had done, this one vibrated a new element. I had no reference point for this energy, and I assumed that it was the energy of an illness I had not encountered before. At the same time, I noticed that as I was describing the nature of her psychological stress, I kept referring to her as having an "inner child" that had never fully matured. I had never used archetypal language before, but as I later reflected on this reading, I realized that my citing the archetype of the inner child contributed more to her understanding of her own nature than anything else I could have said.

After that experience, I welcomed this new energy into my sphere of perception. In each reading following the initial one, more and more impressions of archetypes filtered into the information. I was awestruck by the depth that this material contributed to my understanding of the pattern of a person's conscious and unconscious nature. I was, of course, very familiar with much of what had been written on archetypes in general, such as the work of Carl Jung, but I had never personally encountered this dimension.

I have since come to believe that each of us, while connected to the entire sphere of the archetypal dimension, is simultaneously connected to a personal grouping of twelve archetypes that play a more intimate role in the development and maturation of our psyches. I now refer to this as our Sacred Contract, by which I mean our agreements with the Divine that are continually influencing our conscious patterns of growth. I suspect that we agreed to these contracts in some way, prior to our birth, not through the lens of our personalities but through our souls. For that reason, we cannot fully understand these contracts through the limited sight of our personalities; rather, we must develop an ability to interpret our physical life through its Symbolic meaning. Within that perspective, the physical elements in and of our lives are props on the stage, serving as catalysts that ignite a response from our unconscious minds.

As we enter the age of Aquarius, our unconscious minds are emerging from the depths of the unseen aspects of our being and are stepping more and more into direct contact with our conscious minds. This shift in awareness represents but one of the changes brought about by the approaching energy of the next astrological age. We are obviously meant to continue learning more about ourselves, and the time has come for us to establish direct dialogue with that part of ourselves that has traditionally been called our unconscious.

As with all chakras, the eighth also has its shadow side—or shadow sides. The shadow of the inner child, for example, shows up as the "orphan"—adults with this archetypal pattern believe they were not given the proper parenting as children and so are incomplete as adults. The shadow side of the "prophet" can manifest in the projection of one's own madness as misguided leadership and dark warnings to others. Jim Jones, who convinced a group of followers to commit suicide because of his fearful vision of what was supposedly to come, is one such example. The shadow side of the "mother" archetype is the abusive or negligent mother—a woman incapable of fulfilling the universally accepted role of the loving, caring mother. The shadow side of the "hero" archetype is a chronic workaholic or rescuer.

Archetypal patterns are deeply powerful forces that show themselves within the contents of our dreams as well as within the dramas of our physical lives. I have found that by using the archetypal patterns to interpret the life events of the people with whom I work, I can not only help them dramatically increase their self-awareness but also create an impersonal atmosphere that allows them to observe themselves more dispassionately. The people who have hurt them, and whom they have harmed in some way, are thus lifted to the plane of souls who have played very supportive roles in each other's lives. From this heightened vantage point, similar to the Witness in Vedantic parlance, forgiveness becomes a remarkably easy task.

The Eighth Chakra: Igniting the Fire

Because the eighth chakra connects you to a universal, symbolic dimension of life, to merge with this energy you need to give conscious time to interpreting events and relationships in your life archetypally. I don't mean you should stew in negative juices and dwell on why something didn't work out the way you would have liked. Practice using your Symbolic sight to detach your emotions from a given situation, positive or negative, and observe the details to determine the lesson or guidance they contain. Here are some pointers for using Symbolic sight.

Although Symbolic sight is not an easy art to master, you can begin by controlling how you reflect on a situation. Instead of thinking about it in the first person, describe the circumstances to yourself in a neutral voice. Change "I had an argument with my boss" to "An argument occurred between two people. The cause of the argument was a power play regarding how to perform a task. The state of mind of one of the individuals was obdurate, and that of the other was that of a disciplinarian." One person symbolized a boulder; the other a landslide. This way of detaching allows you to view what is taking place *behind* the physical and emotional surroundings of the event. When you practice viewing situations this way, you will find it much easier to identify the lessons inherent in them and choose an appropriate course of action. Practicing Symbolic sight in conscious, present time will then have a powerful effect on your life and your healing.

Applying Symbolic sight to past events in your life can also help you find the jewel in those experiences. Take some time now to choose a disturbing event from your past and recast it in this detached language. Instead of saying "My father always belittled me whenever I did something he didn't like," say "An adult who was disappointed with his own life chose to compensate by diminishing those around him." Then look at your own life and your actions, and see how you may be creating the same behavior you found so painful in the past.

When you have finished this exercise, whether you are using it for a recent or distant past experience, you can connect with the power of the eighth chakra with the following invocation: "I release all of my illusions, and I accept fully the will of the Divine as the guiding force in my life."

MEDITATION FOR CLEANING OUT THE CHAKRAS

This meditation comes from an American-born devotee and longtime student of Satya Sai Baba who now lives and teaches in India. It should be performed in a quiet area where you will not be disturbed for at least fifteen or twenty minutes.

1. Sit up straight, either in a chair or on the floor, close your eyes, and become aware of the seven chakras through visualization, sensation, or intuition. Visualize, sense, or intuit that the chakras are opening up like camera lenses.

2. Feel or be aware of a golden ball of light, about the size of a basketball, one yard above your head. Feel or be aware of a tan-colored beam or cord of light reaching from your first or root chakra to the center of the earth; this is called the grounding cord.

3. Breathing in a natural rhythm, inhale and feel cosmic energy coming down from the golden ball of light above your head through the seventh chakra, down your spine, and into the root chakra. In the same breath, feel earth energy coming through your feet and up your legs into your root chakra. Allow the two energies to meet, mix, and merge there.

4. Holding your breath only for as long as is comfortable, feel this mixed energy cleaning out the root chakra.

5. Exhale, and let the dirty energy be flushed down the grounding cord into the center of the earth. This has no negative effect on Mother Earth. She burns it in her superheated molten core.

6. Repeat the process, using as many breaths as necessary to clean out the chakra completely. Visualize or sense the chakra from all points of view—up, down, right, left, front, back, in, and out—to be sure it is thoroughly cleansed.

7. When you feel the root chakra is cleaned out, move up to the next one. First, though, begin by once again inhaling and merging the two energies *in the root chakra*. Then, while holding that breath, move the mixed energies to the chakra being cleansed, and work with it there on subsequent breaths. The dirty energy should always be flushed down the grounding cord on each exhalation.

8. If you feel that the energies of a chakra may be influenced by another person in your life, living or dead, surround that chakra with white light to protect it from that influence, which may come in the form of ideas about yourself.

9. The concentration required to do this meditation may build up an energy in the upper body, which may or may not be felt physically but *can* be felt in the form of tension. To relieve this tension, after you have cleaned out all seven chakras, bend forward as far as possible. If you can, touch your forehead to the floor and put the palms of your hands on the floor. (If you are sitting in a chair, just touch your palms to the floor.) Feel the tension energy moving through the top of your head and forehead and through your shoulders and hands into the ground. This is called dumping out. Take some deep breaths and relax until you feel that the tension is completely relieved. Then sit up again and rest with your eyes closed.

10. Now define your space. Begin by getting a sense of the boundary of your aura. It usually extends about fifteen feet from the body.

11. Next, using your mental energy, have a sense of pushing your aura outward until it is about ten yards in radius. Then let it snap back to its natural position, as a stretched rubber band snaps back when released.

12. Now feel as if you are pulling your aura right up against your skin. Then let it spring back to its natural position.

13. Fill your aura with blindingly bright, golden-white light. If you want, you may feel the presence in that light of the deity to whom you feel closest or love the most.

14. Conclude by wrapping your aura in a turquoise light to keep the energy in.

15. Dump out again. Sit up with your eyes closed.

16. After you have finished cleansing the chakras, take a few moments to recall a time, however brief, when you experienced a feeling of transcendence, of being united with everything at once. This need not be a specifically spiritual experience of prayer or meditation but could be a feeling of oneness with the natural world or a fleeting sense of transcending time and space while contemplating a work of art or music, during sexual union, or even an athletic experience. Bring that moment into conscious-ness now and let the energy of that feeling of transcendence per-meate your being, feeling what it is like to be connected at your deepest level to God or infinite vastness. Let yourself feel, if only for half a second, what it is to *become* one with everything.

17. Take what you have received from that experience, and put it into each chakra, going from the bottom to the top.

18. Dump out again. Sit up and open your eyes.

Chapter Eight

◆

USING THE CHAKRAS
AND THE SACRAMENTS
FOR HEALING

At the energetic level, a very real and powerful connection exists between the chakra system as developed in India and the seven sacraments within the Christian faith. Both of these systems can guide us to develop an internal spiritual authority and a consciousness of healing and Divine power.

The connection between the chakra system and other spiritual traditions came to me while I was pondering the nature of truth as a universal force. I noticed, for example, that the teaching that murder and stealing are wrong can be found in every spiritual tradition. On the other hand, teachings about certain dietary practices are unique to specific religions and so cannot be considered universal truths.

Having come to believe in the spiritual authenticity of the chakras, I couldn't help but wonder why the Christian religion, for instance, did not contain a similar teaching. One day, as I was teaching a workshop on intuitive development, I looked at the chakra system that I had drawn on the blackboard, and some part of me projected onto that board the seven Christian sacraments. After the workshop, intrigued and confused, I lined up the sacraments alongside the chakras, in the order in which one would receive them. Gradually, I realized that both systems were illustrating the power of the same dynamic flow of energy that gives life to the human body. I later made a similar connection with the Tree of Life from the Kabbalistic tradition of Judaism, and I saw more and more connections between all three spiritual traditions and understood better their significance to our health.

To test the validity of my ideas, I arranged a workshop based on them. I decided to focus on the sacraments, because the chakra system is still fairly obscure to most Americans, as is the Tree of Life. (Few modern Jews outside the Hasidim still study the Kabbalah, although it is now beginning to enjoy a renaissance.) At first, I considered simply teaching the symbolic meaning of the sacraments and the chakras, but then it occurred to me that in the Christsian tradition, the sacraments are meant to be "taken," so their sacredness can awaken within the human spirit.

This was risky for me, because I am not a priest and so am not ordained—in the traditional meaning of the term—to perform the rituals that coincide with receiving each sacrament. Besides, I thought, the idea of receiving the sacraments might be extremely uncomfortable for many of my workshop participants, who tend to follow spiritual paths completely unrelated to the Christian tradition, or are lapsed Christians with no desire to return to their roots!

As I prepared for this workshop, I asked a dear friend and Episcopalian priest, Rev. Suzanne Fageol, to assist me, explaining that I wanted to present the sacraments in their symbolic rather than their traditional context. The workshop, which took place in Mexico, began with my presentation of the union between the chakra system and the sacraments. The workshop was seven days long, and each daily lecture focused on one chakra, the corresponding sacrament, and the relationship these two forces have to our health and healing. Each evening Suzanne would support my material with her own insights on the sacrament that I discussed during my lecture. Then she would prepare the group to receive the sacrament, if they chose to. Much to our surprise, every member of the group participated in almost all of these holy rituals.

Normally when I give a workshop that lasts for several days, participants tend to bond closely. Yet none of the workshops that I had done in my career compared with what took place in this one. Suzanne and I had hoped that the participants would find the information we were sharing of interest, but neither of us was prepared for the profound spiritual impact it would have on them, or the long-term consequences they would later report. During these sessions, some people healed their emotional and psychological injuries, and in the following months, we received reports of others who had subsequently succeeded at healing their physical illnesses.

I was especially struck by a woman named Sara, who had arrived at the workshop a nervous wreck. At the age of 47, she looked burned out, acted quite neurotic, and seemed to be crying throughout the entire week. She told us that she had worked on her life for years, that nothing had ever helped, and that now she was tired, lonely, and in need of a husband. Frankly, she seemed on the brink of a breakdown, and although she had no single overriding complaint, her condition fit the profile of chronic fatigue syndrome. Sara was Jewish, but she was very interested in our approach to the sacraments, and she took each one with great respect. Each evening—in between bouts of open weeping—she would share some rather remarkable insights she had had that day. She grieved so intensely that it seemed as if she were releasing something much deeper than her present complaints. I don't think I saw her without a Kleenex in her hand all week.

By the end of the workshop, however, Sara looked like a different woman. Within three weeks after leaving, I later learned, she met a man, got engaged the same week, and married him. Sara and her husband both credit that workshop for their marriage. A number of other healings, less dramatic perhaps but no less significant, also took place.

Suzanne and I gave several more weeklong workshops combining the chakras and the sacraments, and they continued to evoke healing energy that impressed and moved us. Although I felt it necessary to have Suzanne, as an ordained priest, give the sacraments formally during these workshops, I do believe that each person alone at home can enact symbolic rituals on their own that will infuse them with the essential energy of these sacraments. Making the right preparations and having the right intention can only magnify that energy. One element that may help more than any other is a home altar or shrine, which you can create somewhere in your house or apartment. It need not be much more than a bridge table or even just a flat piece of wood across two bricks in a corner, where it won't be disturbed. Add a votive candle or two, any image that is meaningful to you—whether Mother Mary, the Buddha, Quan Yin, Jesus, or a parent or spiritual teacher you love and admire—and perhaps a Pyrex or earthenware bowl in which to burn paper, and you're all set.

The rituals that follow, although they may sound simplistic, are actually quite powerful when carried out with a respectful attitude. You may even choose to create a "home workshop" of your own, taking one of the sacraments each week, perhaps on the same day, after preparing for it beforehand. You can take them over a shorter or longer period of time, of course, as long as you allow sufficient time to prepare yourself mentally for each ritual.

THE FIRST CHAKRA—BAPTISM

The first sacrament is Baptism, which represents the introduction of a new life into a family. Through this sacrament, the family accepts responsibility for the physical care of the child, promising before God to give it a home, food, and clothing. Through Baptism, they also commit themselves to teaching this new child about its physical world as interpreted by the family's religion, social outlook, and ethnic heritage. Baptism is thus symbolic of the information that grounds the child to its place on the earth. This sacrament is not connected solely to Christianity—it is an archetypal celebration of the gift of life itself. Its meaning and relationship to the first chakra, which symbolizes our connection to physical life and to groundedness in the energy of the earth, is identical to that of baptismal rituals in other cultures.

By aligning the energy of the first chakra with the ritual of Baptism—think of it as a merger of Symbolic forces—you can begin to look upon your life and family as the environment in which you were spiritually meant to grow up. As difficult as this concept may be for many to handle, accepting it can represent an important first step toward letting go of anger and resentment at wounds inflicted by your family. Childhood wounds are often the most challenging to heal, because by the time we are ready to confront them, many of the people with whom we would like to clear the air have passed on, leaving us only our memories to work with. Still, even the most trying of family environments can eventually be understood as the beginning point of strength.

Despite the fact that many people now accept that they somehow participated in choosing the life into which they incarnated, and that everything about that life is meant to be a spiritual learning experience, they can easily lose sight of this perception in the face of painful childhood memories. The violation you may feel because your family did not provide the emotional and physical support you needed is a wound that penetrates deeply because it is more than a personal wound—it is also an archetypal wound.

The human race knows universally that adults are responsible for their young. This is more than a social responsibility; it is a dictate from Nature herself, providing for the continuity of life. When that "law" is not obeyed, a life current is shattered within the individual. Healing from violations of this law can require effort well into adulthood, because the code of family responsibility to its young reaches into the flow of the life-force itself.

Archetypally, some form of Baptism exists in almost every society. On a Symbolic level Baptism today, reexperienced by adults, whether they were formally baptized or not, offers a perspective that can assist enormously in healing childhood wounds. The Symbolic meaning of Baptism shifts our view of birth from a chance entry into a family to an entry into the spiritual experience of life through the avenue of that family. This archetypal perspective liberates us from the illusion that our lives have been irremediably marked by the quality of our childhood. It also helps us to see that the greater meaning of Baptism resides not so much in our families' acceptance of us as in our acceptance of the whole of our lives as they are, and of the very gift of life itself. It is up to us, as we come to understand what it means to be a conscious individual, to baptize our own lives out of gratitude rather than wait to be baptized by others.

In my first lecture in the workshop in Mexico, I explained that in taking the sacrament of Baptism, the participants were choosing a Symbolic means of transcending the obstacles of their youth and embracing their family and their lives. Seen from that Divine perspective, everyone in their past would seem transformed; they could now see those people as suffering from their own demons or, better still, as their inspiration to walk the path they walk today.

Following this explanation, Suzanne and I offered Baptism to the workshop members as the act of celebrating and accepting responsibility for their own life. Since the workshop was held at a mineral hot springs spa in Rio Caliente, Mexico, we were able to conduct the ritual in a small swimming pool with the hot spring water. Some people stepped fully into the hot natural spring water instead of just having it poured over their head. But each person, as he or she set foot in the water, offered a prayer of thanksgiving for the gift of life. In the privacy of their own hearts, several people later said, they forgave their families and blessed them for having brought them into the world. Grief was shared along with gratitude. At the close, they spoke about their experiences and expresssed the profound belief that this ritual had the power to change their lives permanently.

A woman who plunged—and I mean plunged—into the water, said, "I wanted to poach those memories right out of my body, my mind, and my heart, and by God, I think I did it."

One man remarked that he prayed for grace to start flowing into him because he wanted to see more than just his own life. He wanted to see all the beauty in life and to live consciously in gratitude for being alive.

Another woman later wrote to me that after she returned home, she told her family that she wanted them to understand the meaning of life as a gift instead of the consequence of two people having sex. Her son apparently thought the idea was ridiculous, but her daughter and husband saw the beauty in it, and together they went to their minister and asked him to say aloud the words of the sacrament as he administered it to them. The minister kept insisting that this was not the usual manner in which this sacrament was conducted. "Well," the woman replied, "we're not all that usual either."

One man who had held his family responsible for his struggle with alcoholism and for the way that struggle had "ruined" his life now prayed, as he received the sacrament, that he be given the grace to embrace his family and to release his addiction from alcohol. He later wrote to me that he had not had a drink since.

One woman described the pain of having her daughter tell her she no longer wanted any contact with her. Following this workshop, she wrote to her daughter, sharing with her the Symbolic meaning of Baptism, expressing the hope that her daughter could see the gift of her life from a perspective greater than the connection they shared as mother and daughter. She added that were they never to meet again, she would always be grateful to life itself for the gift of a daughter to cherish. Within six months, they were in communication and on their way to healing their relationship.

One woman said that during the sacrament of Baptism, she felt the energy of life literally illuminating her pelvic region, which was inflamed with infection. She felt light and heat enter into her body, and by the end of the week, the pain of the inflammation had healed.

Finally, one man told me that taking this sacrament had enabled him to release the anger toward his family that he had carried for so many years. He had believed for a long time that this anger could never be healed because none of his family members were alive and so he could not confront them with his feelings. He realized during the ritual that he did not really want to confront them; he wanted to accept them for the people they were. He felt that he had sent them that message through the power of Baptism.

The Ritual of Baptism

Baptism traditionally involves either pouring water over the physical body or immersing the body in water. When you initiate your own baptism, however, your intention should be to cleanse your inner self. To do so, I would suggest that you drink water that you have in some way made sacred: Place some crystals in a container of water and leave it in the sun, or add herbs associated with internal cleansing and let them steep. As you drink this water, hold the intention that you are releasing the toxicity that you associate with your biological family (or any "family" of which you are now a part, including a work family). Be aware that you are in fact accepting and blessing the entirety of your life as it is unfolding in the physical world.

THE SECOND CHAKRA—COMMUNION

The second sacrament is Communion, which symbolically resonates with the meaning of the second chakra. Communion is the sacrament that literally represents the Last Supper, when Jesus said to his disciples, "Do this in memory of me." As a result, Communion now symbolizes the sharing of love and brotherhood with one another. It also represents union with the Divine.

The teaching inherent in all religious traditions that each of us has a Divine spirit within us shines through this sacrament from a Symbolic perspective. Each person with whom we have a union, positive or negative, contains a Divine connection. If breaking bread with them is the physical act of communion, Symbolic Communion is the sharing of energetic "bread" with them. Were we to look upon each other from this perspective, we might well shield ourselves both from the loss of our own energy in confrontations with others and from contamination by negative energy sent in our direction. We would be more prepared to respond to others with kind thoughts rather than negative ones, with the awareness that each of our relationships contains some level of spiritual purpose. This takes a remarkable amount of spiritual discipline, but that is what becoming conscious is all about.

The second chakra energizes our relationships and monitors the quality of energy we exchange with other people. It logs into its data system our consciousness about money, power, and sex—areas of life that involve relationships with other people.

When the second chakra is united with the sacrament of Communion in a positive way, it becomes focused on building healthy, clean, and nonthreatening relationships to money, power, and sex. A sense of safety is always present, giving one the feeling that no matter what problems arise in one's physical life, a way out can be found.

At the Mexican workshop I presented the sacrament of Communion not only as a method of retrieving power but also as a way to prevent the loss of power in future relationships. Symbolically, as we share communion with others, we acknowledge that we are all part of the same spiritual family or source. Moreover, extending the concept of Baptism, we acknowledge that each person in our lives is there for a spiritual purpose, even though we may not be able to perceive it clearly. The spiritual significance of a "negative" relationship may be all but impossible for us to see. Nevertheless, learning to accept that the people who push your buttons in the most annoying fashion are there for a purpose is one effective way of getting back the energy you have invested in maintaining that negative bond. When someone tells me they've found their "soulmate" and it's so wonderful, I say, "No, you haven't! Your real soulmate is the one your body can't stand." Carlos Castaneda once said that we should be grateful to the "little tyrants" in our lives, because they force us to grow and learn more than anyone else does.

I asked the workshop participants to imagine the act of breaking bread with another person from a Symbolic perspective, in which they transfer to another a piece of bread containing the thought-form "I bless you and our interaction, and I ask the same in return." Asking for the same energetic response is appropriate because Communion is the act of sharing. As part of the visualization, I instructed the group to focus on their energy leaving their second chakra and making contact with the other person's second chakra, because this chakra directs our consciousness in terms of our relationships to others.

We may send symbolic pieces of bread containing blessings to others at a distance. We can, and probably should, send them most often to our negative relationships that require healing attention. As you ask for the same blessing in return, visualize the negative energy you have invested in that relationship as healed and returning to your own energetic system. We can also send Communion blessings to people we are scheduled to meet (even if we have already met them) as a way of surrounding that meeting with spiritual energy.

At the Mexican workshop I described the Symbolic meaning of Communion. I told the group that by taking this sacrament, they would actually be taking a vow to try to see that each person has been sent into their lives, as they themselves were sent into the lives of others, for a spiritual purpose. I asked them to take some time to decide whether they really wanted to live within the parameters of this vow. When the time came to receive the sacrament, everyone participated. And once again, following that ritual, people shared their responses.

One man wrote that he had always had a very trying relationship with his boss. They competed constantly for authority in the office and for taking credit for jobs well done. In visualizing his boss as a spiritual companion, he visualized transferring a symbolic piece of bread to him. Afterward he said that while he was uncertain of the influence this ritual was having on his boss, he found that it relieved a great deal of the tension he felt whenever he was near his boss. In the long run, he was fairly certain that his relationship with his boss would change, but he was definite that his own stress level would never again be as toxic.

Another man wrote that he shared the significance of this sacrament with his weekly prayer group. Together they decided to use Communion as a way of healing all those who asked for their prayers. As they prayed, they would image symbolic bread nurturing a person's diseased body and feeding all its tissues with a message. The healthy tissues were told to get stronger, and the diseased tissues were told to "eat of this bread and heal." He reported amazing results that included the healing of cancers in both children and adults.

During the workshop a woman said that she focused her attention on offering Communion to every member of her family as a way of sharing her love and strength with them. This exchange of energy, using a sacrament, made her feel as if God were giving her family a special blessing.

One man especially impressed me by saying that when he received the sacrament of Communion, he visualized God giving it directly to him, and that he intended to use the practice in his life daily. Receiving the sacrament made him feel closer to the Divine than anything he had ever done in his spiritual practice.

The Ritual of Communion

On a piece of paper, write the names of those people with whom you want to share positive energy or with whom negativity has existed. You may also include those for whose safety you wish to pray. Say a prayer of intention: "I place this name on the altar because I am asking for . . ." Even though you perform this ritual alone, you can still break bread, symbolizing your desire to share positive energy with people as a way of sending them grace. You may also say, "It is my intention that the grace I am sending nurture or heal this relationship. I sincerely bless the power of this sacrament to do so." Complete your communion ritual by consuming some of the bread and offering a brief prayer of thanksgiving.

THE THIRD CHAKRA—CONFIRMATION

Confirmation is a universal ritual that represents taking full responsibility for one's actions and living within a code of honor. In the Jewish faith, Bar/Bat Mitzvah conveys the same meaning; within Native American cultures, a vision quest—in which a young man alone in the wilderness undertakes to make contact with his animal spirit—is a ritual of the same caliber. Every society recognizes that there comes a time when their younger members need to announce that they are able to stand alone in this world.

In the West today, we seem to be having a crisis of honor. We have lost the ability to honor ourselves and one another. Lying and deceit dominate politics and public life, academics, business, and even the arts. As a result, our children have virtually no valid role models on which to model their own sense of honor. The complete absence of rites of initiation has only compounded the difficulties for our youth.

Symbolically, Confirmation represents a journey into discovering the real meaning of self-esteem and integrity, the capacity to endure the challenges of physical life and to live according to a personal code of honor. Honor is essential to healing, more essential than we have probably realized. Honor is honesty. It is the promise to oneself above all not to negotiate the boundaries of dignity for material gain. This code of honor, by its very nature, includes keeping one's word, not telling lies, and holding oneself accountable for one's actions. Combining the Symbolic meaning of this sacrament with the third chakra, which represents personal empowerment and self-respect, is yet another natural union of spiritual forces.

I have yet to meet anyone who was born with a strong sense of self-esteem; this form of power must be earned. The lack of healthy self-esteem makes you vulnerable to negative opinions and remarks and subject to the controlling willpower of others; it keeps you in constant doubt about your ability to make decisions for yourself. Furthermore, self-esteem is the root of intuitive ability. Intuition does not come from eating a vegetarian diet or from walking three miles a day while listening to relaxing music on your Walkman. It comes from self-respect and from having the courage to respond to your own thoughts and feelings. The problem is that many people believe somehow that intuition is the ability to see the future. They expect that by developing their intuitive powers and changing their lives accordingly, financial safety and romantic love will await them. Yet intuition is not the ability to see what lies ahead, but the ability to recognize that the disturbances occurring in our minds and bodies are signals telling us that our present situation needs to change—for example, that it is time to quit a job and move on. The door we are seeking will not open until we have taken the initial steps to open it ourselves.

I do not believe that we gain self-esteem, let alone personal empowerment, from reading books and hearing lectures. This is one area of growth that requires you to take risks in the physical world, so that you can learn to rely on yourself. Only by taking risks can we gather power into our bellies, the kind of power that leads to intuition, then to courage. And courage is the energy we need to be able to recognize intuitively the guidance signals that tell us to get on with our lives. Not listening to these signals leads to losing power, self-respect, and ultimately health.

Both the Eastern and Western mystical traditions teach us that when we respect ourselves, personal honor and integrity shine through our eyes. You won't need to tell anyone that you respect yourself; it will resonate from your system. The ability to endure hardships is a matter of spiritual honor, allowing you to receive the energy of respect that pours into your system from others. Giving your word and keeping it, not only to others but also to yourself, is merely an extension of this energy.

At the Mexican workshop, in preparing the group members to receive this sacrament, I instructed them to write down their own honor codes. This was a private act, and they were not to share their honor code with anyone else. Then, in receiving the sacrament of Confirmation, they committed themselves to living a life of honor, integrity, and endurance based upon belief in a God who honors strength.

After this sacrament, a woman told me privately that she was afraid of honor because so much of what she had attained in her life came from acting dishonorably. Although she had never stolen anything, she had engaged in manipulation, exaggeration, and lying. She said that it took a great deal of courage to receive this sacrament because it meant that she would have to live by a standard of behavior that was totally foreign to her. Nevertheless, she was willing to give it a try.

One man laughed and said that writing an honor code made him feel as if he were a Knight of the Round Table—and he loved that feeling. Now, he said, he also felt that he could successfully find the right maiden for himself!

Another man wrote that "living an honorable life is difficult because it limits your choices." His was a particularly precious letter for me, because this man had been a pimp and had thrived on selling stolen goods. But after the workshop he never broke his honor code, no matter how pressured he was by his "former business associates," and he has since built a life for himself that makes him feel proud of who he is.

Of all the many letters I received, I was perhaps most moved by one from a woman who had told us that she suffered numerous health problems and had recently had a hysterectomy. She said that the sacraments of Baptism and Communion really did not mean anything to her, but when she heard the meaning of Confirmation, she sat up and took notice. She had always lived an honorable life, except when it came to herself. She realized that she had always made promises to herself that she did not keep, especially promises to make changes for the sake of her physical body. She had also promised herself that she would finish her education and perhaps join the Peace Corps. Each time she failed in one of these efforts, she lied to herself by telling herself that the time wasn't right or that she simply could not leave her present situation. When she took the sacrament of Confirmation, she finally made a promise to herself that she intended to keep; she promised to follow through on every decision that she made to herself from that day onward. She humorously added that her only way around this was not to use the word *promise* when talking to herself.

The Ritual of Confirmation

Get a journal, and write in it your personal honor code. This will reify what your code actually is, investing it with the aura of a formal contract with yourself, carrying the power of a vow. And the journal will become an ongoing text in which you can write on a regular basis, notating and working through the actions and crises of your life. To start, write down an issue that has the potential to compromise your honor, or an event in which you have already compromised your honor. Then write, "I need guidance on this issue." Now close this sacred book and place it on your altar. Assume that guidance will come, either through a dream or a conversation, or by picking up the right book. But know that it will arrive in your life.

THE FOURTH CHAKRA—MARRIAGE

Everyone knows the literal meaning of the sacrament of Marriage. On a Symbolic level, however, this sacrament involves making loving commitments not to another person but to yourself. Learning to love, honor, and respect yourself, in sickness and in health, until your spirit departs from your body, changes the focus of the sacrament entirely. As we have all heard, unless we can love ourselves, we cannot establish a healthy and supportive relationship with another person.

In learning what it means to love ourselves, most of us go through a stage of narcissism, liberating ourselves from the conventions and codes of society. We all need to go through this phase, because we need to explore the meaning of a spiritual truth within our physical lives. But there comes a point where defining self-love through rebellion and physical indulgence no longer brings satisfaction, and we begin—almost automatically—to love and accept ourselves as we are and face how we understand love and how well we are able to love others. Then we can develop, in our cell tissue, the strength to believe that taking care of ourselves is not an act of selfishness but a necessary spiritual task.

Loving yourself means listening to the messages that come from your heart. Unlike third chakra intuition, which guides us at the physical level, the guidance that comes from the heart speaks to us of the importance of doing only those things that we can "put our hearts" into. Without the support of heart energy, we are internally conflicted, continually trying to silence our inner urgings.

Following our heart leads us to the most fulfilling path we can walk. Yet the heart's voice can be disconcerting because it often threatens the comfortably rational choices we've made with our heads. Many of the women in my workshops have admitted to me, for instance, that their choice of a marriage partner was based more on the physical security that the partner offered them than on any overwhelming emotional or physical attraction. And their decision to stay with the partner long after any feelings of love had evaporated was also based on a concern for security.

Similarly, several men have admitted that they remain in their marriages because of the sense of responsibility they feel toward their children.

Needless to say, the decision to "follow one's heart" in these extremely difficult circumstances is among the most trying choices a person can face in his or her life.

Yet, from a truly spiritual perspective—that is, a place of deep contemplation—a person may come to realize that remaining in these situations contributes not love to others, but the energy of a sad and empty heart. When that is the case, then the individual must confront the decision of whether to leave.

The result of a lack of self-love is continual emotional disharmony. When you are never at peace with yourself, inner tranquillity remains elusive.

None of us needs instruction in how to recognize what our heart is saying. We do need guidance, however, on how to have the courage to follow those feelings, since they will force us to change our lives in any case. But consider the consequences of not listening to the heart's guidance: depression, confusion, and the wretched feeling that we are not on our life's true path, but viewing it from a distance.

Guilt can make learning to love oneself difficult, since many people feel guilty if they take care of themselves before they take care of the people who are dependent on them. No one likes to hear the news that she is no longer first in line, and so we must be strong enough to stand by our newly chosen policy. But the Eastern and Western traditions both teach that the love of oneself is actually a gift to others. The love that flows through your heart purifies not only your own spirit but the love you share with others. Unconditional love becomes a genuine healing force that works for others as well as for yourself. Forgiveness becomes easy, because the damage so often generated by a harsh interaction no longer has the power to bring you to your knees. You can look upon another person with compassion regardless of the degree of difficulty between you. Self-regard conveys the gift of inner tranquillity. This is the teaching of the fourth chakra, completely in union with the Symbolic meaning of Marriage.

Merging this sacrament with the teaching of the fourth chakra to honor ourselves allows passion to wake up within us—not the passion directed toward physical union with another person, but the passion to unleash our own talents or build a different life. This passion allows us to admit what is true about ourselves and to recognize that we may be unhappy living as we are right now. Passion cannot be anesthetized by the logical shenanigans of the mind, because it shuns logic and order, seeking risk as its companion instead. Having a passion for our lives is the true meaning of liberation and self-love.

For my Mexican workshop participants, taking the sacrament of Marriage represented the promise to listen to their heart and to wake up their own passion. Although it sounds magical, once the energy of inner passion is alive and working within you, you must be prepared to act on it. You cannot invite passion into your heart and life and expect it to behave like a polite house guest. Passion can show you parts of yourself that you previously could not imagine. And once you start imagining yourself as the person you could become, you cannot silence the desire to become that person.

Once again, as with all the sacraments, the group in Mexico was instructed beforehand to ponder whether they felt comfortable taking a vow to "love, honor, and respect" the voice of their heart and live according to that voice. Taking this vow is the same as inviting the Divine to give you new instructions on how to live.

Marriage was the sacrament my workshop enjoyed sharing the most, because it lent itself to so many jokes about what their spouses would say when they came home and announced that they had "remarried." In the midst of this lighthearted attitude, I saw people celebrating their own liberation. Naturally, the high they were feeling would diminish once they returned to their home ground, but it was, if only for that evening, absolutely electric.

"I love this idea of loving myself," said one woman. "I work a lot at home, and I'm always receiving faxes. Now I'm going to reply with a message that reads, 'Fax off. I'm on my honeymoon.'"

"Self-love for me feels like a new wind," remarked a woman well into her seventies. "It feels as if I've been given permission to leave everything else behind, and that now it's just God and me."

One man commented that learning to love himself was complicated. As a minister, he was in the business of caring for others, and he was afraid that self-love would cause him to lose his footing because so much of his religious influence was aimed in the opposite direction. He asked if I had any suggestions, and I laughingly replied that he simply change religions. On a more serious note, I told him that this shift in consciousness was going to be hard for everyone, but it might be easier for him if he shared the message with his spiritual community. By so doing, he would grow in his own commitment to this sacrament.

One fireball of a woman remarked that all her life, people had expected her to take care of them. She had eight children and had been happy to nurture them into their adult years, but now it was her time. What made her decision all the more urgent was that she had been feeling her health slipping away, without knowing exactly what the problem was. But in taking this sacrament, she felt she had made a vow that gave her the means to avoid developing an illness.

The Ritual of Marriage

Marriage is traditionally a sacrament in which two people vow to love each other and live the rest of their lives together. When this sacrament is taken by an individual, its meaning must shift to the Symbolic level, as a vow that can be renewed often, as one celebrates an anniversary.

This is one ritual for which you need to prepare in advance. Select from your wardrobe, create, or purchase an item of clothing or an accessory that especially appeals to you, one that represents beauty and love and that reminds you of all that is good about life and yourself. Even fresh flowers or a gift from someone you view as a model of self-appreciation will do. Whatever you choose will represent your vow to appreciate yourself, to take care of yourself, to love and honor yourself in this life. Place the item on your altar, and express your intention to let it serve as a reminder of your own inherent worth.

Whenever you feel the need to nurture yourself, go to your altar and make contact with that item. Remind yourself that you need to be a loving mate for yourself as much as for anyone else. This is a sufficient ritual for the sacrament of Marriage, because above all it is a reminder that care of yourself has to be one of your priorities.

THE FIFTH CHAKRA—CONFESSION

Like marriage, confession is understood in all cultures, because it is universally recognized that the spirit cannot carry its burdens and mistakes without disintegrating. We need to release all that is dark within us lest our psychological and emotional demons consume us and cause us to see all others as dishonest, corrupt, fearful, and guilty of negative actions. When these demons hold sway, we become saturated with the energy of paranoia and are unable to trust others fully.

Today alternative healers often speak about the necessity of "calling our spirits back into our bodies," and they often present this truth as though it were a new concept. Yet the only thing new about it is the language through which we describe it. That language is helpful, of course, because the sacrament of Confession means far more than humbling yourself before another as you admit to doing all the things you should not have done.

Confession is not merely about ruminating about your slip-ups. It demands that you consciously recall the energy of your spirit and direct it into your own being. Many spiritual traditions, along with Christianity, recognize the importance of offering a dying person the opportunity to confess so that the whole of that person's spirit can be released from physical life without leaving fragments behind. Confession requires a supreme act of will-power because it means that you are ready to face your own shadow and to make amends. It is an invitation for justice to come into your life, and even though you may not need to experience justice physically, you are nonetheless recognizing that the choices you make at each moment of your life do indeed have consequences. Even our negative choices directed toward ourselves ultimately cause us to recognize the harm we have inflicted upon ourselves.

As we develop an awareness of our energy, we will be able to tell immediately when it is leaving our body as a result of any negative action, because a part of us instantly clicks into gear, asking us if we really want to act in such a negative manner. We may choose to retrieve our energy in that moment, but if we do not, the body will respond with a sensation that tells us we have just weakened our physical being. This might feel like a rush of guilt through our system, a twinge in the solar plexus (third chakra), or a stirring in our conscience that won't let us rest until we retrieve the energy by rectifying the negative action. Any of these responses indicate that we have misused the energy of our spirit by sending it on a negative mission.

Heightening our awareness of the overall tone of our judgments and understanding the significance of making wise choices, which is the core meaning of the fifth chakra, casts a bright spiritual light on the potential healing force of this energy center. The tranquillity we feel after taking the sacrament of Confession, the sense that we have freed ourselves of darkness, is our signal that the spirit has returned home.

Not surprisingly, no one in my group in Mexico needed to decide whether to take this sacrament. Although Confession is not easy to share in public, the group had bonded so thoroughly by now that their need for privacy was lifted. They also wanted to explore with each other the inner feeling of energy returning to their bodies. "I hope I'm not kidding myself," one woman said afterward, "but I feel lighter than I did before we took this sacrament. Maybe this could be my new diet," she joked.

One man commented that after Confession he felt his body shaking with energy, as if he had been struck by lightning. "As I was taking this sacrament, I prayed that I would never again lie to others. I am ashamed that I have done this in the past, but I actually feel forgiven."

"I've suffered for years with depression," remarked another man. "I have taken drugs to battle it, and I have gone to any number of therapists. I have been diagnosed as manic. I came to the point where I believed that depression was the only state of mind that I would ever have. When you were teaching about Confession, I didn't especially feel that I was guilty of sins such as lying, but I realized that I was always envious of people whose lives seemed to be happier than mine. I don't think that I can change that feeling overnight, but at least now that I know what it is, I feel that I have a way of releasing it."

"I've known that my spirit was not fully in my body ever since I was a child," commented one woman. "I came to understand it more and more as an adult, because that was when I was able to recall that I had been molested as a child—and since recalling those experiences, I have only hated the men who did that to me. I prayed that they would suffer the same way they made me suffer. During this sacrament, I sent them the message that they were no longer in charge of my spirit—I was. And as I did that, I called my spirit back. I hope my feeling that I can finally let go of my childhood is my signal that I will succeed."

The Ritual of Confession

If you burn things externally, they won't burn internally. Take as much conscious time as you need—once a week, perhaps on Sunday—to write down on a piece of paper which of the choices that you've made are negative and will cost you energy. These are choices that don't enhance your life or anyone else's. Then burn the paper in the bowl on your altar, and as the smoke ascends to heaven, say your own prayer asking for greater consciousness so that you don't repeat these negative choices. If you prefer, you can light a candle instead of burning the paper, but still visualize these negative choices dissolving and returning the energy they have wasted to you.

THE SIXTH CHAKRA—ORDINATION

Of all the sacraments, Ordination may be the most difficult to understand at the Symbolic level. As I explained to my workshop participants in Mexico, we are unaccustomed to thinking of ourselves in positive terms, and we measure what is significant in life by its size and how public it is. It is tremendously difficult to break the hold these ideas have on our minds. Although people can grasp the Symbolic meaning of Ordination intellectually, it does not easily penetrate their hearts to engender the passion needed to motivate change.

The path to our own Ordination is one of personal and spiritual development. We can study the meaning of compassion, love, and charity forever without actually practicing them. Just as the preceding sacraments lead us to a deeper understanding of why we need to make spiritual development a priority, Ordination represents a mature opening toward the Divine, to use us as a vehicle for bringing this energy to others.

The original meaning of Ordination involves acts of love and service to others that come naturally through the strength of one's spirit. But when such acts are motivated by weakness, manifesting as the need for recognition and self-gratification, they are contaminated and can actually become a form of seduction rather than contribution. People are easily seduced into believing they are receiving help from another person, particularly when they are desperate for it—which is why unprincipled priests, gurus, and spiritual counselors can so easily take advantage of their students and disciples.

True Ordination can be thought of as the achievement of a very real degree of spiritual maturity, in which the attributes of the spirit shine so clearly that we need not mention they are present—others can see them. Our only task is to maintain these qualities with integrity, which requires that we recognize that they are alive within us.

In my explanation to the group in Mexico, I pointed out that this sacrament embodies a paradox: It emphasizes the necessity of loving and being of service to others in an almost impersonal way. That is, we need not be fully aware of the qualities we have that contain so much power. It is for others to see them in us, and in that recognition they are, in fact, administering the sacrament of Ordination. At the same time, we need to recognize the treasures we are carrying within us. How, you may ask, can we be at once unaware and aware?

Paradox is one of the languages of the Divine. Being unaware of our treasures does not mean we do not see them. It means that we keep our ego in check, in the sense Jesus meant when he said, "When you give alms, do not let your left hand know what your right hand is doing." That does not mean that we banish our ego from our psyche altogether; rather, it means that we maintain a clean ego, one that permits being "in the world but not of the world." We are free to share in the world's abundance, but we must never use our gifts to manipulate that abundance. We can allow ourselves to be loved deeply, but we must never weaken others by the manner in which we love them.

Supporting this position is the energy of the sixth chakra, which represents wise judgment and the true meaning of compassion. Wise judgment is, paradoxically enough, the ability to render no judgment on others but to seek a compassionate understanding of why an individual has become negative or toxic. The application of wisdom carries with it great healing power because it offers guidance without shame or criticism.

Combining the energy inherent in the sacrament of Ordination with the energy of the sixth chakra, which also represents liberation from the power of life's illusions, allows you to see that your greatest contributions to others are often the ones that carry no physical packaging: love, understanding, compassion, joy, optimism, courage, nonjudging, and so many others. Every one of us has the potential to develop these beautiful attributes of the human spirit, and in making such a journey, the healing energy we bring into our lives along the way also heals our own spirit.

Because Ordination is based on the qualities others see in you, I instructed the workshop members to choose the qualities they felt drawn to developing within themselves. In taking this sacrament, they were making a vow to nurture those qualities as a spiritual practice. They would pay attention to how they interacted with others: Were they judging them? Did they want to impress them? Were they seeking recognition from them? What truly motivated them to be of service to others?

These questions cannot be answered overnight. Consequently, Ordination took more processing than any other sacrament for the group members. And because of its association with the priesthood, we instructed the participants to spend the entire afternoon in silence deciding if they wanted to take it at all. Ordination was the only sacrament, in fact, that not everyone decided to take. Because I could see the conflict this particular sacrament was having on them, I wanted to hear after the ritual from those who refrained as well as from those who received the sacrament. Those who did not participate all said, in some way, that they were not prepared to make the personal sacrifices to which such a commitment would bind them. One very honest woman said that perhaps she did not really want to be of such service to others because she was more comfortable receiving assistance than offering it. Another woman said, "I did not take this sacrament because I am not prepared for how it could change my life. I am not ready to consciously release my life to God, because that's how this sacrament feels to me. And even though I know intellectually that I really don't have that much authority over my life, I still need to live in that illusion."

Yet for those who did take this sacrament, their sense of establishing an intimate union with God was evident. They were consciously making a vow to be of service in whatever way God would have them serve. Most important of all, they vowed not to judge their own life's path as insignificant because it might not bear the clothing of physical power. So powerful was this vow that few group members could repeat the words without weeping as Suzanne anointed their foreheads. It became obvious to both Suzanne and me that as each person in turn knelt in faith and trust without fear of God, the unseen power of grace was flowing into them.

"I took this sacrament," one man said, "because I need a focus to my spiritual practice. I need a way to God that speaks not of denying who I am but of delighting in who I am. If this delight emerges and becomes something that can inspire others, fine. If it inspires only me, that's enough, too."

Another man subsequently wrote to me that for him, the sacrament of Ordination was the most powerful one. "This sacrament has given me parameters in which to live and a focus on what is truly important in life. I like believing that the qualities we carry within us, and not the material goods we surround ourselves with, are the significant ones. This idea has given me a great deal of satisfaction."

And one woman who was struggling with breast cancer during the workshop later wrote, "I decided that the quality I would focus on throughout my ordeal with this illness would be inner strength. Instead of dwelling on whether I would heal, I decided to hold on to the belief that regardless of the outcome, I would face it with strength and faith. Much to my surprise, after my surgery to have the tumor removed, I woke up in my hospital bed knowing that not only was the cancer fully removed from my body, but I would also be given many more years to live."

The Ritual of Ordination

This ritual can apply either to your daily work, whatever it may be, or to a specific task that has been handed to you or that you've agreed to take on. By ordaining your work, you acknowledge that it is sacred work, whether it consists of making art or emptying bedpans, running a household or running a corporation. If you view your work as sacred, you're more likely to do your best and avoid shoddy efforts. You can ordain any task and make it sacred, so that it represents the original meaning of Ordination, which is to recognize that you are specifically suited for this task.

Once again, you may want to prepare some water in a special way by placing some crystals or aromatherapy oils in it to energize it, the way a priest blesses holy water. Write the name of your job on a piece of paper, and place it on your home altar. Or if you prefer, anoint your desk, the tools of your trade, your computer, or any item that represents your desire to do in an honorable way what you have been ordained to do. While anointing, hold the intention to make your work sacred.

THE SEVENTH CHAKRA— EXTREME UNCTION

The sacrament of Extreme Unction, or last rites, is traditionally given to a person who is preparing to die. Its significance lies in the sick person's acceptance of leaving behind the possessions of his or her life, both physical and emotional.

Extreme Unction is normally administered only once, but from a Symbolic perspective, in the realm of our own thoughts and feelings, it can be administered once a day, because it signifies our desire to release the unnecessary baggage we carry with us. It represents the release of all that is dead in our lives, and our conscious choice not to use our life-force to keep alive that which has passed from us. More than the others, this sacrament offers us a discipline through which we can live in the present moment.

While it may be uncomfortable at first to think of the past as "dead," this is nonetheless an accurate description of the place we call "yesterday." Breathing our life-force into keeping the past alive is like choosing to live in a mausoleum. It is cold and dark, and the dead do not speak to us.

We are not meant to carry the past within us as if it were still alive. What is over is over, and using our energy to fuel events or relationships long gone is like breathing life into a corpse in hopes of a resurrection. The cost of such actions to both the body and spirit is enormous. In explaining the Symbolic meaning of Extreme Unction to the group in Mexico, I presented it as a means of consciously releasing, even on a daily basis, everything that they no longer wanted to carry with them in their energy. Unlike the sacrament of Confession, which releases the negativity one is carrying, Extreme Unction is directed toward recognizing that phases of your life have passed on. The end of your youth, the death of your marriage, the closure of a relationship, entering retirement, leaving behind the home you once lived in— all of these are examples of life stages that continually change and eventually are no longer a part of who and what we are today.

People hold on to these life stages in many ways—even cosmetically, with surgery that attempts to lift the years from our face and body. We need to ask ourselves if our desire to be who and what we once were, and to have what we once had, contributes to our health or endangers it. The answer ought to be so evident that I don't have to say it. Baggage from the past does not keep the tissue in our body alive—how can it? We have only so much energy with which to run our lives, and using that energy to run our past more than our present causes us to run into energetic debt. Eventually the resources with which we pay this debt come from the energy in our cell tissue, weakening our body into a condition that allows illness to develop.

The inherent energy of Extreme Unction combined with the energy of the seventh chakra, which represents our connection to eternity and the Divine, celebrates the truth that all that was good about our past remains alive within us and around us, and that what is dead needs to be dead. We cannot fully feel the grace that assures us of our own immortality if we continue to fear and fight the passage of years. This is a paradox of our own creation and not one that heaven has designed for our empowerment.

Our connection to the eternal force of the Divine through this sacrament includes all we have been, all that we are, and all that we are meant to become. This connection is a promise that our life-force is endless and that we can transcend any obstacle. Releasing yesterday through a greater understanding of our Divine nature is the pathway to rising above all that has happened to us on the physical plane. Along the way, we reach for the spiritual truth that physical events are nothing more than illusions and that the physical manner in which they manifested in our lives is meaningless.

Healing can be thought of as a way to teach us to live in the "here and now." Although Christianity has been guilty of placing too much emphasis on the afterlife, the Gospels themselves speak of letting go of the past and of striving to live in the present moment. Jesus remarked to the disciple who wanted to return home to bury his father, "Let the dead bury their own dead" (Matthew 8:22). Likewise, the Eastern traditions teach us that the physical world is nothing more than illusion and that living in the present moment is what matters.

Few members of the workshop needed time to decide whether they wanted to participate in the ritual of Extreme Unction. It was almost as if they were ready to dump the contents of their emotional suitcases on the floor, as a symbolic release of everything they no longer wanted to carry with them. "I have been ready to let go of so many things for so long," remarked one woman, "but I have always felt so guilty about that. And now I feel that this is what God intended, and that feels so good to me."

One man commented, "I have always felt that my background was my identity. I now realize how foolish that is, and I will work to let go of that part of myself."

I later received a letter from a woman who wrote, "I have always wanted to sell my childhood home, which I inherited from my parents. They told me to take care of it because it was all they had, so I have hung on to that place despite its being an emotional and financial burden. Well, now, I'm pleased to say, that place is up for sale."

And one man phoned me, saying, "I have been ill for a long time with various ailments. I've had chronic pain, lower backaches—all kinds of things. Since practicing this visualization about letting go, I started to have the thought that I was carrying everything on my back. I now believe that I'm going to finally get out of this pain, and I believe it is due to my continual practice of this sacrament."

The Ritual of Extreme Unction

Begin by asking yourself, How much energy is draining from me? How much of the dead am I carrying with me in my daily life? On a piece of paper, write down whatever dead weight of the past you feel you are lugging around with you. Put the paper in a Pyrex or earthenware bowl on your altar, and light a match to it. As it goes up in flame, visualize yourself dissolving the bonds that have tied you to the incident or incidents, and allow your energy to return to you. If you prefer, find a small object symbolic of the event— for a car accident, say, a small toy car will do—and anoint it with the holy water you have prepared. Say a prayer in which you release your energy from the event symbolized by that object. It can be as simple as saying, "I don't want this in my life anymore."

As you feel your energy returning, say a brief prayer of thanksgiving.

Epilogue:
Snow White and
the Seven Chakras

◆

Over the past few years, following in the footsteps of Carl Jung and Joseph Campbell, a number of gifted teachers and Jungian analysts, notably Clarissa Pinkola Estés, have reinterpreted some familiar myths and fairy tales. I've always been impressed by their work but never thought of applying this technique myself until I happened to be watching the Walt Disney version of *Snow White and the Seven Dwarfs* on television one day. I wouldn't normally expect Walt Disney to be the conveyor of Symbolic truth, so what I saw crept up on me by surprise, and of course speaks to the power of the original fairy tale. It is also an ultimate story of healing and spiritual awakening.

The Queen is standing in front of the mirror—the archetypal signature of the self, which in the Disney version happens to be surrounded by the signs of the zodiac. The Queen asks, "Mirror, mirror, on the wall, who's the fairest of them all?" And the mirror answers, "Snow White."

Perhaps Snow White is the symbol of the Queen's higher self, and the Queen the traditional ego, attached to materialism and control. The Queen is really saying that she has to kill her higher self because it's causing her to notice things she'd rather ignore. Her higher self, after all, is scrubbing the floors of the castle, which represents the whole of the self, like a true mystic who sees God in everything and finds peace and fulfillment in the most mundane tasks.

The Queen orders her huntsman to kill Snow White and bring back her heart—the middle chakra that unites higher and lower self! We think we're hitting on something new by finally attaching our biology to emotions, but it's no accident that the physical heart has always been associated, both in myth and popular jargon, with truth and love, the very elements that make up the fourth chakra.

Instead of killing Snow White, of course, the huntsman allows her to escape into the forest, and he kills a pig and brings *its* heart to the Queen. Snow White then begins her dark night of the soul, spends the night in the forest, frightened of all the eyes around her. But by dawn, she realizes that the eyes were those of animals that were protecting her. Having made it safely through the dark night, she sets out on a journey and comes upon a bridge leading to a thatched hut. She crosses the bridge—the classic symbol of spiritual transformation—and enters the house of her new self. She immediately starts to clean it out and reorder everything in it according to her own lights. The Queen, her lower self, has been overcome.

The Seven Dwarfs, who are miners, present themselves, but Snow White has them wash before they can come in. In other words, upon discovering her chakras, she immediately sets out to purify them. In the Indian tradition of Kundalini Yoga, adepts set out to cleanse and purify the chakras from the bottom up so that the sacred energy of the life-force that lies coiled at the base of the spine can rise up through the crown of the head. That purification can be accomplished gradually through prayer and meditation, or in some cases it may happen in a flash, spontaneously. In any case, it is the prelude to an opening of the soul.

Meanwhile, back at the castle, the Queen discovers that her higher self is still alive. She gets a poisoned apple—the traditional forbidden fruit of knowledge of good and evil, although it is never mentioned by name in the Book of Genesis. The Queen gives the apple to Snow White to eat, whereupon Snow White falls into a deep sleep. As she sleeps, she descends into the underworld of the archetypal realm. To emerge from this archetypal slumber, she has to merge her animus and anima, the prince and princess, the male and female components of her soul. Out of that merger comes the resurrection of a whole being, conscious self-understanding, and healing.

Our goal is much the same as Snow White's—to get our ego to stop fighting our higher self, to unify the elements of our nature, to make friends with our seven chakras, and to wake up and take charge of our lives. The difficult parts of the journey— wandering through the dark night, purifying our energy centers, descending into the deepest reaches of our psyches—are the keys to the challenge of healing. It goes without saying that not every healing crisis will have a "fairy-tale ending," but every effort you make, regardless of how insignificant it may seem to you, will always bring you closer to a state of spiritual and physical health.

Acknowledgments

✦

First and foremost, I am eternally grateful to my brilliant editor and dear friend, Leslie Meredith, for all of her faith in me and in this material. To Chip Gibson, publisher of Harmony Books, my deepest thanks for all of your support. And to Andrew Stuart, Leslie's assistant editor, my deepest thanks.

As always, I remain thankful to my agent, Ned Leavitt, who has guided me through a thousand storms while remaining a steady and wise force in my life—all my love, Ned.

Some special thanks to Peter Occhiogrosso, without whose assistance this manuscript would never have been completed. Peter's task was monumental; the reorganization and editing of this entire manuscript in record time. Throughout this ordeal, Peter remained calm and supportive when I needed it most. For me, Peter was a life-saver, not to mention a book-saver, and I shall remain ever appreciative for his contribution to this book and to my life. And to Janet Biehl, the copy editor of this manuscript, my thanks.

And to Tami Simon, founder of Sounds True Productions, I want to express more than gratitude. Tami first produced the basic material on "Why People Don't Heal" on audiotape a few years ago. Her faith and support in my work—and in me—has given me the desire to bring this information all the more into the public arena because of the response of that first tape. I will never be able to express to Tami—and to the staff of Sounds True—how much I appreciate all they have done for me.

M. A. Bjorkmon and Rae Baskin, founders of the Conference Works, have been the backbone support team for the majority of my workshops and for the growing interest in my work; I treasure my bond with you.

As always, personal friends and family form the core support group to a person. And for me that core begins with the love of my mother, my brother Ed, sister-in-law Amy, and my cousins Marilyn, Mitchell, Chris, and Ritchie, and to my incredible friends, Norm, Suzanne, Jim G., and Virginia Slayton—who started me on my teaching career. Mary Neville and Paula Daleo stand alone in this category because not only are they my assistants, they are "forever friends" without whose help and guidance, my work would be even more confused than it already is.

And finally, I am grateful to the "gods" for having sent Donald into my life just at the right time. He helps me realize more each day the essential message of this book—that love is the most significant force in life, not to mention the most beautiful.

Caroline Myss

Index

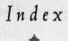

About the Author

✦

Caroline Myss, Ph.D., is the author of the best-selling *Anatomy of the Spirit* and a pioneer and international lecturer in the fields of energy medicine and human consciousness. Her work is also featured in two PBS videos, *Why People Don't Heal* and *The 3 Levels of Power,* available through Unapix Entertainment. Since 1982 she has worked as a medical intuitive: one who "sees" illness in a patient's body by intuitive means. She specializes in assisting people in understanding the emotional, psychological, and physical reasons why their bodies develop illness. She has also worked with Dr. C. Norman Shealy, M.D., Ph.D., founder of the American Holistic Medical Association, in teaching intuitive diagnosis. Together they wrote *The Creation of Health: Merging Traditional Medicine with Intuitive Diagnosis.* She lives in Oak Park, Illinois.

Why People Don't Heal and How They Can is available on videocassette. Also available on videocassette by Caroline Myss is *Three Levels of Power and How to Use Them.*

To place an order for your own videocassette copy, or to recieve a Unapix Entertainment catalog, please contact:

Unapix/Miramar
200 2nd Avenue West
Seattle, WA 98119
(206) 284-4700
(206) 286-4433

e-mail: miramar@usa.net
http://www.uspan.com/miramar